Treating Obesity in Primary Care

Angela Golden

Treating Obesity in Primary Care

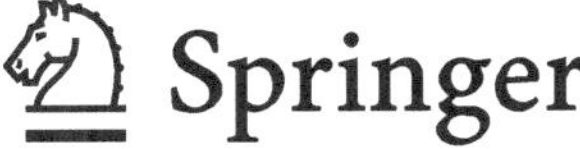

Angela Golden
NP from Home, LLC
Munds Park, AZ
USA

ISBN 978-3-030-48682-2 ISBN 978-3-030-48683-9 (eBook)
https://doi.org/10.1007/978-3-030-48683-9

This Springer imprint is published by the registered company Springer Nature Switzerland AG
The registered company address is: Gewerbestrasse 11, 6330 Cham, Switzerland

Thanks to Mike, you have supported me in every adventure I have decided to go on—and writing this book was an adventure!

To all my patients and the colleagues that have supported me in learning to treat obesity—thank you for the honor of knowing you and please keep teaching me.

And to my mom, dad, sibs, sons, daughters-in-law, and grandchildren, your love and never-ending faith in me kept me supported.

Preface

To best treat obesity, the clinician must first understand the environment the patient has experienced in receiving healthcare and clearly recognize the underpinnings of obesity as a disease. The pathophysiology of the disease and its complications can help guide treatment.

Evaluating obesity in the chronic disease model will provide primary care with a structure that is familiar to clinical practice. The details of using evidence-based practice recommendations with the foundational components of the obesity treatment plan; eating plans, physical activity, and behavioral interventions will be covered. Then reviewing the supportive treatment of medication and/or surgeries, procedures and devices.

After completing the education on obesity as a disease and current treatment options, the next step is putting this into practice in a busy primary care clinic. Several examples of how this can be accomplished have been provided, including billing information, so that the practice can be paid for the work being done.

Munds Park, AZ, USA Angela Golden

Contents

Part II Building a Treatment Plan

Author Bio

Golden

is a current Fellow and past President of the American Association of Nurse Practitioners (AANP). She received her doctoral degree from Arizona State University in 2008. Dr. Golden has been certified as a Family Nurse Practitioner through the AANP–Certification Program since 1998. Her tenure as the President of AANP gives her a unique outlook on the nation's perspective of healthcare. She owns NP Obesity Treatment Clinic where she provides evidence-based obesity treatment. She earned OMA's Certificate of Advanced Education in Obesity Management and the Specialist Certification of Obesity Professional Education, an internationally recognized certification.

Dr. Golden has a great deal of experience as a consultant in the development of patient education materials, has authored a book and a chapter on obesity management, written several peer-reviewed articles, participated in research, and been interviewed by lay media on obesity treatment. She presents nationally and internationally with an emphasis on obesity, health policy, leadership, and clinical care.

Introduction

I sit down to write this book after several years of hearing from my colleagues that they understand obesity is a disease and it needs to be treated but they talk about how much is expected of them in primary care and how can they be expected to do to add ONE MORE THING. My goal is to help each provider (or clinician) in a primary care practice understand:

- Importance of the disease
- How to treat this disease from an evidence-based perspective
- How to create a blueprint for integrating this into a busy practice

There is another reason I am writing this book. I am a person with obesity. I have the disease controlled or in maintenance, but it requires daily attention. My father died from this disease in 2009. This is a personal and passionate project for me.

The book will cover what obesity is, why and how it impacts the body, and then go through the treatment plan or process. Finally, using case studies, I will demonstrate the "putting it all together" and how this can be added into a primary care clinic.

I would like to say that the ideal way of treating obesity is in multidisciplinary teams, just like we read about diabetes and hyperlipidemia or any chronic care model. However, at the end of the day, not all of us have the luxury of all of the disciplines and access to multidisciplinary teams in our primary care practices as described in the literature. So, throughout the book, I will primarily talk about the treatment occurring in primary care and make note of other disciplines that can be part of the care you can utilize through referrals for the care of your patients with obesity. Thank you for caring enough about your patients with obesity to select this book.

For so many years, obesity was seen as a simple calculation of calories consumed and not enough energy expended. Research has taken us well beyond this answer about the disease. The endocrine society says "…growing evidence indicates that obesity pathogenesis involves processes far more complex than the passive accumulation of excess calories" [1]. Looking at the incidence of obesity prevalence in the USA, the Center for Disease Control and Prevention in 2016 showed 39.8% of adults affect by it, this is 93.3 million people with the disease of obesity [2]. Thirty percent more adults have preobesity (overweight) classification. No state has lower than 20% rate of obesity anymore. These numbers alone explain why all of us in primary care must embrace the treatment to the chronic disease of obesity. But if this isn't enough reason, projections estimate that by the year 2030 over 85% of adults will be affected by obesity or preobesity. Worldwide, the World Health Organization (WHO) shows obesity rates have tripled since 1975 [3]. In 2016, 1.9 billion adults had preobesity while 650 million had obesity. The global economic cost of obesity is 2 trillion dollars, contributing to the global GDP. This is as much as what is spent on armed conflicts and smoking combined! [4]

Obesity was once considered a problem for only high-income countries but is now on the rise in low- and middle-income countries. Even in Africa where so much under nutrition occurs, obesity is on the rise. On top of this, the WHO says obesity and overweight are linked to more deaths than underweight. This information demonstrates the urgency our healthcare system needs to have to treat obesity.

Key Points

1. Rates of obesity and preobesity are progressing.
2. Primary care providers must begin to take responsibility for treatment of the chronic disease of obesity.
3. Obesity is more complex than calories consumed and energy expended.

Disclaimer

1. The goal of this book is to provide you with the most relevant and current information on treating obesity and then how to implement this information in primary care. Additional prescribing information for each medication can be found at the healthcare provider sites for each medication. This information is not a substitute for further education and staying up to date.
2. The book has been thoroughly researched and evaluated for accuracy. Clinical practice is a constantly changing process and new information becomes available every day. Each provider is responsible to consult additional resources and apply information to their clinical practice as appropriate in addition to this book.
3. NP from Home, LLC disclaims any liability, loss, injury, or damage incurred as a consequence, directly or indirectly, of the use and application of any of the contents of this book.

References

1. Schwartz M, Seeley R, Zeltser L, Drewnowski A, Ravussin E, Redman M, et al. Obesity pathogenesis: an endocrine society scientific statement. Endocr Rev. https://doi.org/10.1210/er.2017-00111.
2. Center for Disease Control. 2020. https://www.cdc.gov/obesity/data/adult.html. Accessed 10 Apr 2020.

3. World Health Organization. 2020. https://www.who.int/newsroom/fact-sheets/detail/obesity-and-overweight. Accessed 10 Apr 2020.
4. Swinburn BA, Kraak VI, Allender S, Atkins VJ, Baker PI, et al. The global syndemic of obesity, undernutrition, and climate change: the Lancet Commission report. Lancet. 2019. https://doi.org/10.1016/S0140-6736(18)32822-8.

Part I
Understanding the Disease

To best treat obesity the clinician must first understand the environment the patient has experienced in receiving health-care and clearly recognize the underpinnings of obesity as a disease, the pathophysiology and how it causes complications.

Chapter 1
Bias and Stigma Related to Patients with Obesity

PUT YOUR EAR DOWN NEXT TO YOUR SOUL AND LISTEN HARD.

ANNE SEXTON

Introduction

This chapter examines how bias and stigma impact patients with obesity specifically in relation to healthcare. Explanations of bias and stigma will be discussed. The perspective of barriers and how to overcome these are reviewed. Creating a safe environment for patients with obesity is critical to providing treatment.

Key Reason
To treat obesity for any patient, that patient must first feel safe in your clinic. Bias and stigma around obesity are real and prevent many people with obesity from reaching out to their healthcare provider. This chapter will discuss the reality of bias and stigma and how you can avoid this being a barrier in your practice.

A. Golden, *Treating Obesity in Primary Care*,
https://doi.org/10.1007/978-3-030-48683-9_1

Bias

One of the reasons that obesity starts its treatment much differently than we do with hypertension or diabetes is the sensitive issue that our patients have faced about their weight. Because of this it is important for us to approach the patient with obesity a bit differently than we would a patient with diabetes. After all, if a patient came into your office with an HgBA1C of 13, you wouldn't ask the patient's permission to talk about that, you would just go ahead and explain what the number meant and what treatment is needed to be instituted. But with obesity we must take into consideration the experience that our patients have had with stigma and bias in healthcare. So it's important for us to approach them with nonjudgmental, non-blaming language and demonstrate empathy. What does that even look like. Details of approaches are discussed more in the behavior chapter. The 5As for obesity guides our treatment and starts with ask. Ask the patient's permission to talk about their weight and obesity. Prepare for this and script it out so you aren't hesitant. Hesitancy might imply something you didn't mean.

As we consider the issues of bias, let's look at an example that can be found on the Internet, the word "obesity." A Google search for the phrase "people with autism" you get roughly seven times more results than for the phrase "autistic people." The same is true for asthma and diabetes. However, when searching for obesity it is 12 times more likely to get results for obese versus obesity (see Table 1.1). The word obese is more a label than a disease or condition thus being equal to bias and discrimination. We must be sure that our language is not shaming or biased as we talk with patients, and we need to find ways to make obesity part of our normal language of healthcare, just as we do for other chronic dis-

Table 1.1 Definition of bias and stigma

Bias	Prejudice in favor or against one thing
Stigma	A mark of disgrace associated with circumstance, quality, or person

eases. My personal experience with bias/stigma was a visit to a cardiologist; as he was leaving the room, literally he had his hand on the doorknob, he pointed at me and said "you need to eat less and exercise more" than walked out. And he charted he had discussed my weight with me. It didn't feel much like a discussion, and this is minor compared to what I hear from many patients with obesity. My dad's experience, and keep in mind he had severe obesity, was at many different providers' visits; he would be asked, "do you have diabetes," he would say no, and every provider he ever saw would say, "really, I'm surprised." They never talked about the 350+ pounds on his 5′8″ frame.

It's very important that you have that 30 second elevator speech ready to go when our screening tool of the BMI demonstrates that further conversation is needed. The Strategies to Overcome and Prevent Obesity Alliance also has a discussion tool for providers. Many studies, including the ACTION study in which I got to take part, show that patients want us to discuss their weight and provide them with guidance [1]. When we don't bring it up, we actually are giving them a message of stigma and bias. After all, if they had elevated glucose or an elevated blood pressure, we definitely would be bringing that up. From the patient's perspective why are we not bringing up their weight. After all, those of us with obesity – it is obvious, we have to wear it.

Research has shown that formally diagnosing the patient who has overweight with complications or obesity is a strong predictor for success in treatment of obesity [2]. The United States Preventive Services Task Force (USPSTF) now has guidelines that recommend intensive behavioral interventions for any patient with a BMI ≥ 30 kg/m^2.

Eat less and move more as counseling does not in any way approach the complexity of the disease, nor does it move us toward a productive conversation with our patients. Each of us needs to understand the complexity of this disease so that when we have the discussion with patients we are coming from a physiologic perspective of an endocrine disorder. Now don't get me wrong, I'm not suggesting that by asking to discuss obesity is what changes the patient's ability to lose weight and treat obesity. But how we start this conversation allows the patient to know that they have a partner in the treatment of obesity. Many patients do not see their healthcare provider as the person that can help them lose weight. Almost every magazine and celebrity has an answer to their problem. The average number of times the patient has made attempts to lose weight is somewhere between five and eight depending on the research [1]. And patients never understand why they can lose the weight successfully and yet the weight seems to always come back. As part of the education we all need to be very aware how weight regain occurs and the underlying pathophysiology that causes the weight regain. Patients fell like a failure and have their own blaming language in their heads. The discussion about the physiology of weight regain can be a step to removing their own self-blame. Another thing that can help patients really see obesity as a disease process is to do a weight and obesity history just like we would for other chronic diseases. I think it's pretty clear why we should be the ones discussing this disease with our patients. But how do we do that in a compassionate and blameless way (Table 1.2).

Table 1.2 Sample questions to "ask"

Looking at your vital signs I see your blood pressure is good (or well controlled) but your BMI is elevated. This is one of the measures for a disease called obesity. Can we talk about this today or make an appointment to talk about this soon? (notice this gives the patient more control but isn't a yes or no answer – is a when answer)
I see on your chart that your weight is (has been) elevated for a while. I would like to work with you to treat this. Would today be a good time for us to talk? (notice here, if I get a negative answer, I left the door open)
Can we talk about your weight and how it impacts your life and health? I would like to share with you information about evidence-based treatment and how we can partner in this treatment (this statement asks permission but before I take a breath, I want the patient to know I will be with them and that there are treatments)

Barriers

Most Common Barriers from the Provider: Time, Billing, Education

What I hear from providers as their primary barrier is a lack of time; I have to ask "do you make the time if your patient comes in with a blood pressure of 170/100, or an HgBA1C of 8.9." The answer is "of course." Yet both of those diseases are *complications* of obesity. So the real barrier isn't having enough time, it is how to add "one more thing" to an already packed day. Every practice recognizes the percentage of patients with elevated BMI, but we are unsure of a process to approach obesity. To break this barrier, understanding that obesity is a cause of so many of the diseases we are treating demonstrates that obesity has to rise to the top of the problem list.

Another barrier for treating obesity is being told we can't get reimbursement for obesity. There are many providers in insurance-based practices, family, internal medicine, or specialty practices that are getting paid. The billing chapter provides more details.

I hear from providers all the time that they just don't have the education about obesity from their primary educational programs and they don't have the tools to do the education. The purpose of this book is to bring all that information into one place to provide the information and the application for treating obesity.

Office Issues

- The next day you go to work or if you are at work right now stop reading and go look around your office.
- Start in the waiting room. Is your office welcoming
- Do you have high capacity chairs both in the waiting area and in your exam room?

- What does the reading material look like, is there only the latest magazines promoting quick weight loss or are the reading materials promoting healthy lifestyles?
- Office equipment
  - Look at your scale, how high does the scale go, is it in a private weighing area?
  - Do you have large size blood pressure cuffs, extra-large gowns, longer needles for blood draws, and/or large speculum?
  - Does the exam bed have assistance device to get on the table, what is the weight limit?
- Bathroom
  - Do you have pedestal toilets versus wall-mounted?

All of these things and a few more can make your practice look welcoming to patients who have obesity (as well as be safe). The Rudd Center for Food Policy and Obesity has a wonderful resource you can use in your practice [3].

Now that you have done a visual inspection of your practice and made note of anything that needs changed, you can move to the staff in your office. Assure every employee in the office, from the front desk to the person bringing the patient into the exam room, understands the disease of obesity and the weight bias that many of our patients have experienced. It's very important to have your own language so you are comfortable with the patients and your colleagues. Patients will recognize your comfort with the disease based on your language. So, can you explain how obesity is a disease in a way that patients can understand? Can you explain obesity as a disease to professional peers? If you can do both of those things, it will be much easier to have the conversation with the people who buy equipment, your peers, and your patients.

Keeping in mind our patients' experience of stigma and bias makes it easier to understand why we have to start the conversation differently than we would if we were talking about other chronic diseases (Table 1.3). Different people have different ways to approach this, but often it can be approached because of the reason the patient is there to be

TABLE 1.3 Starting that conversation

I encourage you to write your own script but here are some examples from my practice (many adapted from http://stopobesityalliance.org/wp-content/themes/stopobesityalliance/pdfs/STOP-Provider-Discussion-Tool.pdf)
"Susan, I am so glad you are here today for your well visit. I see in the chart that your weight has increased over the past few years. Could we talk about this? There are new treatments for the disease of obesity that may benefit you."
"Hi Mark, it is great you are here today for your blood pressure check and updated visit. We have gone over your labs I would like to review your vital signs as well. One of the measurements shows that it could be impacting your elevated blood pressure. That measurement is your weight. Could we talk about how that can be treated?"
"Martha, before we finish your visit today, I noticed that your weight is increasing. This can be unhealthy for you and may be a part of your knee pain. If you are interested, we can talk about this and I can show you treatment options and we could create a plan of action together."

seen. An example is a patient is there with diabetes, and their BMI is 33. You can bring up the fact that their diabetes could be improved through treatment of their weight. And then ask if it would be okay to discuss that with them. Very few patients will say no, they've been waiting for you to bring it up. In my primary care practice, when I ask them in the same breath, I tell them that I have treatment approaches that can help them. In those few instances when the patient does not want to talk about the weight, I let them know that's fine today but let's make an appointment to talk about it soon. And I reiterate that there are treatment strategies to help them be successful in treating the complications of obesity as well.

Once we start the conversation, the first thing I do is actually talk about obesity as a disease. I want them to see that it's an endocrine disorder very similar to diabetes, especially if they have diabetes or they have a family history of diabetes, this seems to help bring it into perspective. I also ask questions about their readiness and what their support systems look like. There are many communication strategies that can be used and most of us have used motivational interviewing in many situations, from smoking cessation to helping patients deal with other diseases.

Another acronym to use for a communication strategy: FRAMES [4] (Table 1.4).

Table 1.4 FRAMES – communication strategy

F	feedback	I think the key here is the word respectful. Before talking about unhealthy behaviors, it's important for the individual to understand that you're there to help them overcome those behaviors, or work through them
R	responsibility	The patient should understand that they will have a large role to play in this treatment plan. Be careful that they don't think you're blaming them or being disrespectful but they still need to understand that this is a partnership not a one-way street
A	advice	As with any time you're helping a patient with education, it's important that what you're saying is clear and direct. This should only be given in combination with understanding where the patients coming from. For instance, giving advice on eating plans, but not first determining at what the patient is currently eating and isn't very respectful. Providing an overview of available eating plans and letting the patient select the plan they feel they could best adhere to offer an opening for the discussion.
M	menu	Using the example I gave about the different eating plans is providing the patient with the menu of options. It is allowing the patient to be part of the decision-making process.

TABLE 1.4 (continued)

E	empathy	This starts with what your practice looks like. In the waiting room, look again at the chairs and reading material. These are the first thing the patient will see and can speak volumes to the patient and actually is the start of the communication. Does the providers nonverbal communication match the verbal communication?
S	self-efficacy	Healthcare providers telling the patient the options go along way based on research. It is important for us to instill confidence and optimism for the patient. In practice that means that we are looking for their successes even if they're small. Example is the patient who's eating out 10 times a week, the goal was for five times a week, but the patient only managed eight times a week. That still has to be looked at as a win; it's a 20% reduction in eating out at fast food places.

Practice Pearls

- Patients with obesity have experienced tremendous bias and stigma in healthcare settings.
- Evaluate your own possible bias, consider taking the Harvard Implicit Bias evaluation regarding weight: https://implicit.harvard.edu/implicit/Study?tid=-1
- Listen to the patient and be empathetic; this will go a long way toward building a relationship the patient trusts and can provide a good base for continuing treatment.
- Find your personal language for discussing obesity and treatment with weight loss.

References

1. Kaplan LM, Golden A, Jinnett K, Kolotkin RL, Kyle TK, Look M, et al. Perceptions of barriers to effective obesity care: results from the national ACTION study. Obesity. 2016;26:61. https://doi.org/10.1002/oby.22054.
2. Yaemsiri S, Slining MM, Agarwal SK. Perceived weight status, overweight diagnosis, and weight control among US adults: the NHANES 2003-2008 study. Int J Obes (Lond). 2011;35(8):1063–70.
3. Rudd Center. Checklist for assessing. http://www.uconnruddcenter.org/resources/bias_toolkit/toolkit/Module-4/4-02ChecklistForAssessing.pdf. Accessed 10 Apr 2020.
4. Searight HR. Realistic approaches to counseling in the office setting. Am Fam Physician. 2009;79(4):277–84.

Chapter 2
Obesity as a Disease

THINGS THAT MATTER MOST MUST NEVER BE AT THE MERCY OF THINGS THAT MATTER LEAST.

JOHAN WOLFGANG VAN GOETHE

Introduction

This chapter examines the complexity of obesity as a disease including genetic, environmental, and behavioral factors. Chronic disease model is described and then discussed in relation to obesity. Diagnosing obesity is examined with appropriate methods for primary care. The importance of recognizing and diagnosing obesity as a disease directly impacts the approach to treatment of obesity.

Key Reason
We must recognize obesity as a disease in order to understand the treatment paradigm. This chapter will discuss the reason to classify obesity as a disease and appropriate methods for diagnosis in primary care.

A. Golden, *Treating Obesity in Primary Care*,
https://doi.org/10.1007/978-3-030-48683-9_2

So Is Obesity Really a Serious Chronic Disease?

Over 250 years ago, Dr. Malcolm Flemyng is quoted as saying "Corpulency, when in an extraordinary degree, may be reckoned as a disease, as it in some measure obstructs the free exercise of the animal functions; and hath a tendency to shorten life, by paving the way to dangerous distempers" [1]. The rationale for obesity as a chronic disease is twofold. First obesity itself can impact a person directly (e.g., forces on joints), but it is also the underlying cause of other diseases that have been well established (e.g., diabetes and hyperlipidemia).

Obesity is a disease in this author's opinion because genetic, environmental, and behavioral factors contribute to the following:

- The underlying pathophysiology
- Dysfunction of the neuroendocrine regulation of appetite and energy function
- Increase in morbidity and mortality
- Impairments in physical and physiological function

It was not until 2013 that the American Medical Association recognized obesity as a disease through their house of delegates [2]. The AMA decision was likely a more political one as they debated this on the floor of the house of delegates after the scientific committee approved the request to have it named a disease. The AMA has criteria to determine if they will label something as a disease [3]. The disease must show impairment of normal functions and harm or morbidity. Obesity met impairment of normal functions through physical and physiologic impairments such as inflammation, insulin resistance, dyslipidemia, as well as the impairment in satiety regulation in the hypothalamus. The characteristic signs and symptoms they considered included increase in body fat mass, impaired mobility, low self-esteem, and altered metabolism. The final characteristic of harm or morbidity as noted by the AMA was met due to obesity-related complications such as cardiovascular disease, type II diabetes, metabolic syndrome, cancers, and early death [2].

Many organizations have been arguing for decades about whether or not obesity is a disease. In 2004, the Centers for Medicare and Medicaid Services (CMS) removed the language that obesity was not a disease. Prior to the AMA declaration, The Obesity Society, Obesity Medicine Association, American Association of Clinical Endocrinologists, and Endocrine Society, to name but a few, were already publishing about obesity as a disease. Shortly after the 2013 AMA declaration of obesity as a disease, many other organizations followed with their own statements. A sample of organizations include American Academy of Family Physicians, American College of Cardiology, American College of Surgeons, American Society for Reproductive Medicine, and American Urological Association. Additionally, the World Health Organization, Federal Drug Administration, and National Institutes of Health have recognized obesity as a disease. In 2015, the Nagoya Declaration was passed at the 8th Asia Oceania Conference to recognize obesity as a disease.

Definition of a Chronic Disease

A chronic disease is one that causes the entire body, an organ, or system to malfunction over time. It has stages and end organ dysfunction and causes other diseases. The disease is manifested by signs and symptoms.

Obesity as a Chronic Disease

The Obesity Society uses this definition to describe how obesity is a disease (Table 2.1) [4]. Obesity has structural abnormalities such as left ventricular hypertrophy, ectopic fat deposits, lymphedema, and excess or enlarged adipose tissue. The signs and symptoms of obesity include insulin resistance, dyslipidemia, chronic inflammation, and urinary incontinence. Examples of signs and symptoms include hyperphagia, and in severe disease, hypoventilation syndrome and exercise intolerance occur. Finally, obesity has been associated with 236 other conditions and is clearly a positive cause for many

TABLE 2.1 Definitions of obesity

World Health Organization	Abnormal or excessive fat accumulation that presents a risk to health. A crude population measure of obesity is the body mass index (BMI), a person's weight (in kilograms) divided by the square of his or her height (in metres). A person with a BMI of 30 or more is generally considered obese. A person with a BMI equal to or more than 25 is considered overweight Obesity (and overweight) are risk factors for common chronic diseases (examples: diabetes, cardiovascular diseases and cancer). Once considered a problem only in high income countries, overweight and obesity are now dramatically on the rise in low- and middle-income countries, particularly in urban settings [15]
AACE/ACE	A chronic disease characterized by pathophysiological processes that result in increased adipose tissue mass and which can result in increased morbidity and mortality [16]
OMA	A chronic, relapsing, multifactorial, neurobehavioral disease, wherein an increase in body fat promotes adipose tissue dysfunction and abnormal fat mass physical forces, resulting in adverse metabolic, biomechanical, and psychosocial health consequences [17]
CDC	Weight that is higher than what is considered as a healthy weight for a given height is described as overweight or obese. Body Mass Index, or BMI, is used as a screening tool for overweight or obesity [18]. Obesity is a complex health issue to address
	Obesity results from a combination of causes and contributing factors, including individual factors such as behavior and genetics. Behaviors can include dietary patterns, physical activity, inactivity, medication use, and other exposures. Additional contributing factors in our society include the food and physical activity environment, education and skills, and food marketing and promotion
	Obesity is a serious concern because it is associated with poorer mental health outcomes, reduced quality of life, and the leading causes of death in the U.S. and worldwide, including diabetes, heart disease, stroke, and some types of cancer [19]

Table 2.1 (continued)

TOS	Obesity is a multi-causal chronic disease recognized across the life-span resulting from long-term positive energy balance with development of excess adiposity that over time leads to structural abnormalities, physiological derangements, and functional impairments. The disease of obesity increases the risk of developing other chronic diseases and is associated with premature mortality. As with other chronic diseases, obesity is distinguished by multiple phenotypes, clinical presentations, and treatment responses [20]
WOF	Obesity is a medical condition described as excess body weight in the form of fat. When accumulated, this fat can lead to severe health impairments. The prevalence of obesity across the world continues to rise, and this is now recognised as one of the most important public health problems facing the world today [21]

chronic conditions such as diabetes, hypertension, hyperlipidemia, and Non-Alcoholic Fatty Liver Disease (NAFLD) [5]. The Obesity Medicine Association uses sick fat, obesity-related complications, and the relapsing multifactorial causes to define obesity as a disease [6].

The World Obesity Federation (WOF) goes further in their definition saying we must look at the larger public health perspective of the environment as part of our definition and causation in order to control the obesity epidemic. It goes as far as to say the early detection and treatment of childhood obesity should be considered similar to vaccinations – an absolute must. Dr. Bray is quoted as saying, "… continuous effort is needed to control obesity because it is a relapsing disease process" [7] (p720).

WOF says obesity is a disease by using an epidemiologic approach. This is different than any other organization. In this model they list the primary issue being that of an environmental agent (with food the main agent). A secondary issue around the world being decreasing levels of physical activity. However, they're not saying eat less and move more as the total solution. They discuss endocrine disrupters, including epigenetic changes, certain medications, and the decline in smoking rates. Their model also takes into account that some people are more susceptible to the environmental agents. Hundreds of genes have some association with the disease of obesity [7].

Obesity is a dance or interaction between our genes, the environment, and our behavior. One of the arguments for obesity as a disease is the malfunction of the hypothalamus that regulates food intake and hunger. Additionally, the infiltration of adipose cells into other organs and the amount of inflammatory marker secretion from adipose tissue add to the evidence of obesity as a disease. The inflammation likely underlies the altered metabolism. *Obesity is not a lifestyle choice.* Very few people with obesity have not tried to self-treat it. Surveys of people with obesity (PwO) have shown 60% say they have tried to lose weight in the past year [8]. This is not to say that making behavioral changes is not needed in the treatment. But it needs to be directed changes and not the billions of dollars spent on the next magic pill, remedy, or exercise program to "melt" off the fat. Unfortunately, our own healthcare colleagues are part of this deception targeting patients with obesity.

Why Do We Care if Obesity Is a Disease?

So that's all well and good justifying obesity as a disease, but is this of any real importance in clinical practice? The Obesity Society recommends that all societies and associations recognize obesity as a chronic disease for several reasons [9].

1. To advance funding for research. The funding will provide the understanding of this complex disease.
2. Assisting the public in perceiving obesity as a disease. Many continue to see obesity as a lifestyle choice or willpower behavior. This is causing tremendous bias and stigma and preventing PwOs from utilizing healthcare for treatment.
3. To stop unscientific and inappropriate weight loss claims.
4. Allow healthcare systems and academic institutions educating the providers to ensure the appropriate education is occurring.

5. Financial coverage for evidence-based obesity treatment. As it stands now many insurers have obesity as an opt in for employers. This is the only chronic disease as an opt in feature.

Does Obesity Need to Be Treated?

When reviews from the NHANES study look at people with obesity, there's a clear association and an increase in morbidity and mortality rates [10]. Tremendous number of research articles have now shown that obesity on its own is associated with an increase in cardiovascular morbidity and mortality, as well as greater all-cause mortality. Dr. Hamdy says in the Medscape review; "obesity is indisputably the greatest preventable health-related cause of mortality after cigarette smoking" [11]. One example used to demonstrate the serious consequences of this disease is the patient relative risk for coronary heart disease. If the patient has a BMI < 30 kg/m^2 but ≥ 25 kg/m^2, studies show risk of 1.72, while a BMI ≥ 33 kg/m^2, there's a relative of risk 3.44 [11]. So now that we all agree obesity is the disease and that it needs to be treated, how is it diagnosed?

Diagnosis

BMI is the first step, but it is really a screening tool (see BMI chart). In most cases we need more than BMI. As we will see in the pathophysiology section visceral adiposity holds the greatest risk for pathology, so waist circumference can be used as a marker for adiposity in the visceral area. In primary care these two data points are the easiest from a number's perspective. In a conversation with Dr. Lee Kaplan (November 2019), he stated, "Neither of these are the perfect way to diagnose obesity. The future will bring more accurate methods and will need to be integrated just as we have with DEXA scans for bone density." Dr. Kaplan is the 2019–2020 president of The Obesity Society. He is also the director of the Obesity, Metabolism and Nutrition Institute, founding director of the Weight Center at the Massachusetts General Hospital, and associate professor of medicine at Harvard Medical School.

BMI requires a measured height, not stated. This is going to require a possible change in how your support staff does vital signs. You will likely also need to teach support staff how to measure the waist circumference.

As we know BMI is a measurement of overall mass so someone with a great deal of muscle could have a higher than "normal" BMI yet have very low body fat percentage. Additionally, on the other end of this is the person with a normal BMI but still has an increased percentage of body fat, called sarcopenic obesity. Sarcopenic obesity is often found in geriatric population.

The process for doing a waist circumference should be done in all patients with a BMI ≥ 25 kg/m^2 if of non-Asian descent and ≥ 23 kg/m^2 if the patient is of Asian descent. It is done by finding the top of the iliac crest with a tape measure parallel to the floor and not compressing the skin (Fig. 2.1). Be sure to complete the measurement at the end of normal expiration. Greater than 40 inches in men is a measurement of concern and greater than 35 inches in women. In people of Asian descent, the waist circumference is 35 inches for men and 31.5 inches in women. People of Asian descent have more total adipose tissue and visceral fat and therefore may be at higher risk of developing type 2 diabetes for a given BMI than whites [12].

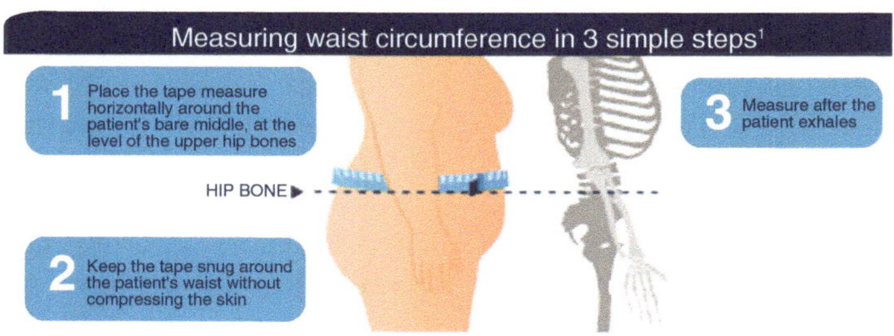

Figure 2.1 Measuring waist circumference

The concept of waist circumference to help diagnose obesity comes from the National Cholesterol Education Program (NCEP) Adult Treatment Panel 3 based on their definition of metabolic syndrome. NCEP found an increase in CV risk with a waist circumference greater than 102 cm (40″) in men and 88 cm (35″) in women. NCEP also looked at waist to hip ratio greater than 0.95 in men, and greater than 0.8 for women with higher risk for complications [13].

There are other ways that adiposity can be measured and therefore used to diagnose obesity (Table 2.2). Skin fold is frequently done in health clubs but is the least accurate method so is not recommended in primary care. Bioimpendence scales provide a measurement more than weight with body fat percentage, muscle mass, and water. The scales are based on electrical resistance conducted through the body components. Lean body tissues, which contain body fluids and electrolytes, are highly conductive, low resistance electrical pathways. Skin, bone, and adipose tissue, on the other hand, are very poor conductors and offer increased resistance. The technology provides an estimated total body water, and using this value of TBW, there is an estimate of

TABLE 2.2 Pros and cons of measuring for obesity diagnoses

Method	Pros	Cons
Body composition scales	Accurate	Expensive Hydration dependent Most insurances – not reimbursable
CT/MRI	Extremely accurate in determining subcutaneous and visceral adipose tissue	Expensive Not all machines can accommodate patient with severe obesity
DEXA	Extremely accurate in measuring fat mass, non-bone lean mass, as well as the usual bone mineral content	Somewhat expensive Not all machines can accommodate patient with severe disease Rarely reimbursable from insurance

free-fat mass and body fat or adiposity. Some machines provide information about the amount of adipose on tissue in various compartments.

CT and MRI scans can be used to accurately determine the adipose tissue in visceral areas as well as deposited in organs. The current standard technique for measuring visceral adipose tissue volume is a single cross-sectional image at L4 and L5 levels. The accuracy is within 1% margin of error. Obviously, both of these are very expensive, and with 70% of Americans having increased BMI as their screening numbers, this is not reasonable. Researchers and obesity practice centers may use BodPods or underwater weighing but again due to cost and time are unlikely to be helpful to those of us treating this in primary care. Dual energy radiographic absorptiometry (DEXA) is used primarily by researchers to look for fat mass and free fat mass but may be a cost-effective way in the future to diagnosis and monitor patients.

Staging Obesity

Now that we have a diagnosis, the next step is to stage the disease. This can help us in primary care and decide how assertive to be with treatment. Very much like hypertension, a patient with a mild elevation of blood pressure may be given lifestyle treatment and then if this is not effective medications. One difference with obesity is the vast majority of our patients have been attempting lifestyle interventions for years and that should be taken into consideration.

The WHO stages obesity based solely on the BMI (Table 2.3). Of course, the problem with this is that BMI doesn't identify the amount of adiposity.

AACE and Edmonton Obesity Scale take staging further using obesity-related complications and comorbidities as part of their staging system. AACE has a three-stage system (Table 2.4). EOSS has a five-stage system taking into account medical, mental, and functional information. Stage 0 has no signs or symptoms of obesity in any of the parameters, while Stage 4 is end stage in all parameters.

Table 2.3 WHO staging system for obesity

Grade or stage	BMI (kg/m^2)
1	25–29.9
2	30–39.9
3	BMI $\geq$ 40

Table 2.4 AACE staging system for obesity

Grade or stage	BMI	Complications
0	$\geq$25 kg/m^2 to 29.9 kg/m^2 or BMI $\geq$ 30 kg/m^2	No identified complications. Stage 2 has. BMI is still $\geq$25 kg/m^2
1	$\geq$25 kg/m^2	Has one or more mild-to-moderate complications that can be treated effectively by treating obesity
2	$\geq$25 kg/m^2	At least one severe complication and may require more aggressive treatment

Is It Even Important to Make a Diagnosis or Can Just Treating the Complications Be Enough?

Studies have found patients who received a formal diagnosis of overweight or obesity from the healthcare provider to be successful [14]. This is one reason why it is so important to be sure that the patient understands the diagnosis (Table 2.5).

Practice Pearls

- Obesity is a disease due to its chronic nature and causation of other diseases.
- Assure appropriate diagnosis beyond BMI.
- Acknowledge that patients with a diagnosis are more likely to get treatment.

TABLE 2.5 BMI ranges

BMI	Non-Asian descent (kg/m²)	Asian descent (kg/m²)
Underweight	<19	<18.5
Normal	20.0–24.9	18.5–23.0
Pre-obesity/ overweight	25–29.9	23–27.5
Obesity	≥30	≥27.5

References

1. Bray GA. Obesity is a chronic, relapsing neurochemical disease. Int J Obes. 2004;28:34–8.
2. Kyle TK, Dhurandhar EJ, Allison DB. Regarding obesity as a disease: evolving policies and their implications. Endocrinol Metab Clin N Am. 2016;45(3):511–20. https://doi.org/10.1016/j.ecl.2016.04.004.
3. American Medical Association. How diseases get defined and why it matters. 2018. https://www.ama-assn.org/delivering-care/ethics/how-diseases-get-defined-and-why-it-matters. Accessed 10 Apr 2020.
4. Jastreboff AM, Kotz CM, Kahan S, Kelly AS, Heymsfield SB. Obesity as a disease: the Obesity Society 2018 position statement. Obesity. 2019;27:7–9.
5. Yeun M, Earle R, Kadambi N, Brancale J, Lui D, Kahan S, Kaplan L. A systematic review and evaluation of current evidence reveals 236 obesity-associated disorders (ObAD). Poster presented at: Obesity Week Conference of the Obesity Society. New Orleans; 2016.
6. Obesity Medicine Association. What is obesity? n.d. https://obesitymedicine.org/what-is-obesity/. Accessed 10 Apr 2020.
7. Bray GA, Kim KK, Wilding JPH, World Obesity Federation. Obesity: a chronic relapsing progressive disease process. A position statement of the World Obesity Federation. Obes Rev. 2017;18(7):715–23. (Bray, 2017, page 720).
8. Martin CB, Herrick KA, Sarafrazi N, Ogden C. Attempts to lose weight among adults in the United States, 2013–3016. NCHS Data Brief, No. 313. Atlanta: Centers for Disease Control and Prevention; 2018.

9. Jastreboff AM, Kotz CM, Kahan S, Kelly AS, Heymsfield SB. Obesity as a disease: the Obesity Society 2018 position statement. Obesity. 2018;27:7–9.
10. Hruby A, Hu FB. The epidemiology of obesity: a big picture. PharmacoEconomics. 2015;33(7):673–89. https://doi.org/10.1007/s40273-014-0243-x.
11. Hamdy O. Obesity. Medscape. 2018. https://emedicine.medscape.com/article/123702-overview. Accessed 10 Apr 2020.
12. Chinese Community Health Resource Center. n.d. https://www.cchrchealth.org/health_calculators_p/body-mass-index-bmi-for-adults/. Accessed 10 Apr 2020.
13. Christian A, Mochari H, Mosca L. Waist circumference, body mass index, and their association with cardiometabolic and global risk. J Cardiometab Syndr. 2009;4(1):12–9. https://doi.org/10.1111/j.1559-4572.2008.00029.x.
14. Kaplan LM, Golden A, Jinnett K, Kolotkin RL, Kyle TK, Look M, et al. Perceptions of barriers to effective obesity care: results from the national ACTION study. Obesity. 2016;26:61. https://doi.org/10.1002/oby.22054.
15. World Health Organization. Obesity. n.d. https://www.who.int/topics/obesity/en/. Accessed 12 Apr 2020.
16. American Association of Clinical Endocrinologists. Treatment algorithm for the medical care of patients with obesity. 2016. https://www.aace.com/disease-state-resources/nutrition-and-obesity/treatment-algorithms/treatment-algorithm-medical-care. Accessed 11 Apr 2020.
17. Obesity Medicine Association. Definition of obesity. 2017. https://obesitymedicine.org/definition-of-obesity/.
18. Centers for Disease Control and Prevention. Defining adult overweight and obesity. 2020. https://www.cdc.gov/obesity/adult/defining.html.
19. Centers for Disease Control and Prevention. Adult obesity causes & consequences. 2020. https://www.cdc.gov/obesity/adult/causes.html.
20. Jastreboff AM, Kotz CM, Kahan AS, Heymsfield SB. Obesity as a disease: the obesity society 2018 position statement. Obesity. 2018;27:7. https://doi.org/10.1002/oby.22378.
21. World Obesity Federation. About obesity. n.d. https://www.worldobesity.org/about/about-obesity.

Chapter 3
Physiology of Adipose Tissue

THERE IS AN ART TO CLEARING AWAY THE CLUTTER AND FOCUSING ON WHAT MATTERS. IT JUST REQUIRES THE COURAGE TO TAKE A DIFFERENT APPROACH.

GEORGE ANDERS

Introduction

This chapter examines the role of appetite and satiety regulation in the state of homeostasis. The regulation of appetite and satiety is a complex feedback mechanism within the brain and various hormones. Adipose tissue is the most prevalent tissue in the body. It helps regulate body energy homeostasis, temperature, reproduction, glucose balance, and immune system. Understanding the physiology is critical to recognize the pathophysiology of the disease of obesity.

Key Reason
For obesity to make sense as a disease there must first be an understanding of the physiology of appetite and satiety regulation. The purpose of adipose tissue also needs to be clarified. The importance of understanding the physiology is the impact on understanding pathophysiology and the targets of

A. Golden, *Treating Obesity in Primary Care*,
https://doi.org/10.1007/978-3-030-48683-9_3

treatment. This chapter will discuss the physiology of appetite and adiposity.

The complexity of appetite and satiety regulation is well beyond eating food. Hunger, or appetite, is the adaptive response to the need for higher energy levels for cellular metabolism. Homeostatic mechanisms involved in promoting and inhibiting feeding behavior have been studied and include gut hormones (e.g., ghrelin, cholecystokinin, insulin, and leptin) and neural activity in relevant brain regions. Environmental cues, cognitive, reward, and emotional factors play an important role in food intake which may override homeostatic requirements [1].

The modulation of food intake is typically integrated to maintain a constant weight status, and defective integration produces obesity or excessive leanness. To adapt to daily variations in energy balance, our bodies sense and integrate information about energy availability that is conveyed to the brain by peripheral hormones (examples, pancreatic polypeptide (PP), cholecystokinin (CCK), peptide YY (PYY) and nutrients like glucose, free fatty acids (FFA), and amino acids (AA). These molecules regulate feeding behavior by acting on neurons in the hypothalamus and the brainstem. The gut itself responds to food resulting in the release of incretins (examples, glucagon-like peptide-1 (GLP-1) and gastric inhibitory polypeptide (GIP)) and insulin, as part of this regulatory process [2].

Central Nervous System Control of Eating

There are some experts that believe obesity is a brain disease because the hypothalamus is thought to have homeostatic control of eating (more on the hormones impacting this in a few minutes). It does this through a complex feedback mechanism primarily in the arcuate nucleus. These neurons express various transmitters that respond to the peripheral hormonal signals increasing appetite and decreasing energy expenditure or decreasing appetite and increasing energy expenditure. The thalamus, midbrain, and striatum impact cognitive control or influence our eating behaviors. This includes reward, emotional, and memory signals. For most of our lives food has served as a reward or substitute to emotions. "Eat this you will feel better, less fearful, less unhappy, less mad, etc." (See Figs. 3.1 and 3.2.)

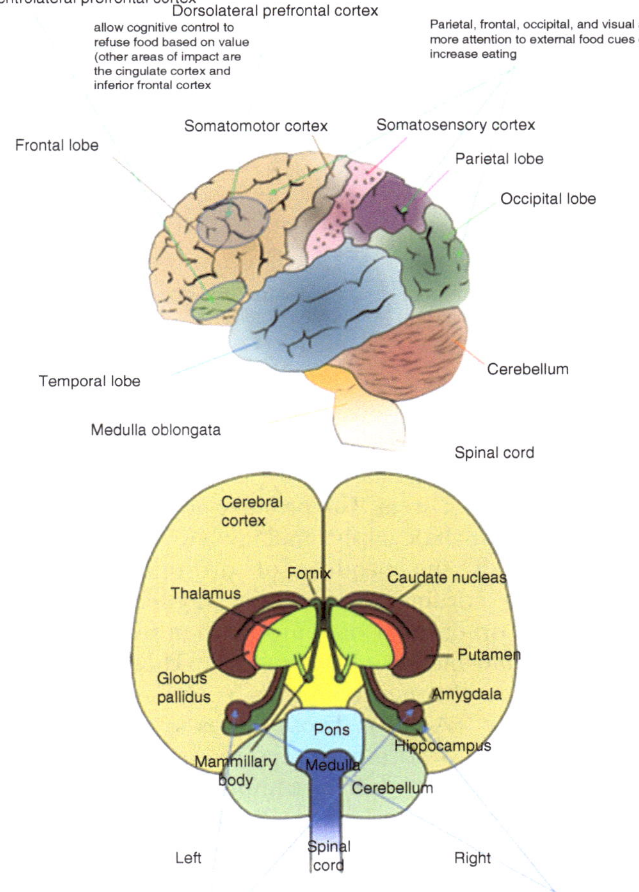

FIGURE 3.1 Brain areas of appetite

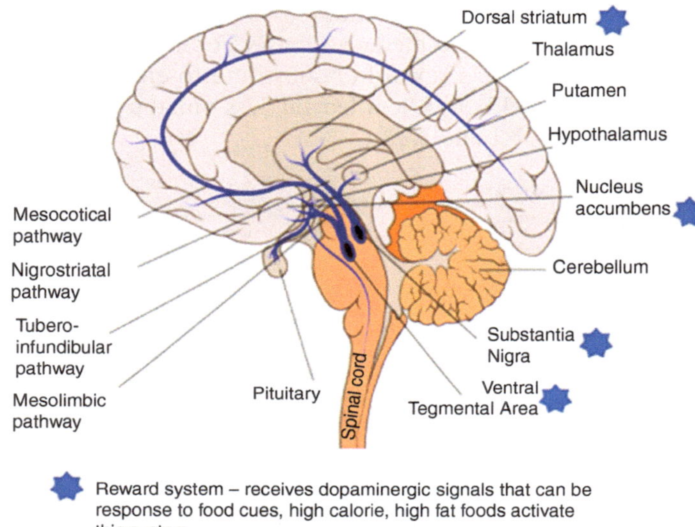

FIGURE 3.1 (continued)

The arcuate nucleus has two types of neurons that project into other brain areas. The primary neurotransmitters of these neurons include alpha melanocyte stimulating hormone, which is the product of pro-opiomelanocortin (POMC) and cocaine-amphetamine-regulated transcript (CART). The other types of neurons when stimulated illicit food intake and increased bodyweight. These neurotransmitters include the neuropeptide Y (NPY) and agouti-related peptide (AgRP). Those areas of the brain are governed by the GI hormones secreted in response to food entering the GI tract. As an example, CCK is secreted in response to lipids entering the duodenum. This acts on receptors that transmit a signal to the brain via the vagus nerve contributing to satiation [3].

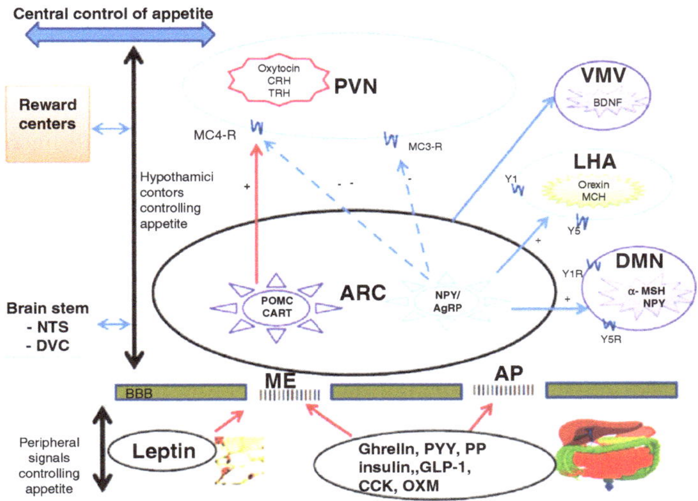

Figure 3.2 CNS control of eating. Short and long signals for food intake control. Abbreviations: ARC arcuate nucleus, NPY/AgRP neuropeptide Y and agouti-related peptide, POMC/CART proopiomelanocortin and cocaine- and amphetamine-regulated transcript, PVN paraventricular nucleus, LHA lateral hypothalamic area, DMN dorsomedial nucleus, VMN ventromedial hypothalamic nucleus, ME median eminence, AP area postrema, GLP-1 glucagon-like peptide-1, CCK cholecystokinin, PP pancreatic polypeptide, PYY peptide YY, OXM oxyntomodulin, BBB blood-brain barrier, MCH melanin-concentrating hormone, α-MSH alpha melanocyte stimulating hormone, BDNRF brain-derived neurotrophic factor, CRH corticotrophin releasing hormone, NTS nucleus tractus solitaries, DVC dorsal vagal complex, TRH thyroid releasing hormone, MC4-R melanocortin 4 receptor, MC3-R melanocortin 3 receptor, Y1R and Y5R neuropeptide Y receptors 1 and 5

Physiology of Adipose Tissue

Adipose tissue used to be thought of as having only three purposes: storage of extra energy to be used as fuel later, shock absorber around vital organs, and under the skin to help with body heat insulation and production. Adipose tissue is the most prevalent tissue in the human body. It is not all bad; it actually has numerous functions including the regulation of total body energy homeostasis, temperature regulation, reproduction, glucose balance, and even a role in our immune system.

Adipocytes start as mesenchymal stem cells. Adipose cells first become fibroblasts, and through a process using peroxisome proliferator-activated receptor gamma (PPAR-γ) they differentiate to pre-adipocytes and then to mature adipocytes. PPAR-γ can be stimulated by environmental factors, for instance, obesogenic medications as well as by human adenovirus–36. There are other factors that promote adipocytes maturation; insulin, growth factors, and glucocorticoids are promoters of this maturation. The sympathetic nervous system, on the other hand, inhibits adipocyte proliferation. This occurs through the effect of adrenergic receptor and a suppression of lipolysis. This clearly explains how beta blockers have adverse side effects of weight gain.

There are three types of adipocytes: white, brown, and beige. White adipocytes are used to store lipids and then release fatty acids when our cells need energy. This type of adipocyte can be found in the visceral compartment and subcutaneously. It is through the sympathetic nervous system and the binding of epinephrine and norepinephrine on the white adipocyte beta-adrenergic receptors that lipids are released. Brown adipocytes are found primarily in the cervical and subclavicular areas of the body. Because they are rich in mitochondria, which puts out energy, they're involved in non-shivering thermogenesis for heat production. Brown adipocytes are found in greater proportion in infants and young children than in adults. There has been some research showing that adults with obesity have lower amounts of brown adipose tissue than those of normal weight. Beige adipose tissue is found among white adipocytes. This cell seems to have a lot of mitochondria and thermogenic capacity. And under certain external stimuli white adipocytes can be transformed into beige. Examples of the external stimuli include chronic exposure to cold, long-term therapy with PPAR-γ agonist, such as pioglitazone, and/or products of exercise (irisin and lactate).

But wait … that's not all. Adipose tissue plays a role in endocrine function. Adipose tissue secretes factors for immunologic responses, impacts the vascular system, and helps appetite regulation.

Leptin is a hormone made and secreted by mature adipocytes. Leptin is known for its effect on satiety in the brain, impacting food intake and body weight regulation. But did you know it also plays a role in fertility and hematopoiesis. Adipose tissue is a site for estrogen biosynthesis and steroid hormone storage.

Adipose tissue secretes other peptides, cytokines, and compliment factors (Table 3.1). Part of these secretions help regulate adipocyte metabolism and growth and play an important function in endocrine signaling to regulate energy homeostasis.

Adipocytes are incredibly active. They release protein and lipids, and this is the only organ with unlimited growth poten-

Table 3.1 Cytokines and proteins

Adipocyte proinflammatoy cytokines
Alpha 1 acid glycoprotein
Serum amyloid A
C-reactive protein homolog pentrazin-3
Lipocalin 24p3
Adipocyte-specific proteins
Adipsin (complement factor D)
Adiponectin resistin
Acylation-stimulating protein
Visfatin
Retinol binding protein-4

tial throughout life. The communication tool for these cells are adipokines. Adiponectin is an adipokine that impacts insulin use in the liver, decreasing gluconeogenesis. Adiponectin has been shown to promote synthesis of HDL cholesterol and antagonizes fat deposition in the liver. There are proteins that play a role during transcription in the control of adipogenesis, and the three most studied at this point are cytosine-cytosine adenosine-adenosine-thymidine (CCAT)/enhancer, C-EPB gene family, and PPAR-$\gamma\gamma$.

Adipocyte cells expand in size as they deal with triglyceride and then divide when they reach their maximum size, which is how it is the organ that can expand and enlarge. If the body needs energy, a lipase enzyme inside adipose cells releases glycerol and fatty acids from the breakdown of triglycerides into the blood which are available for energy to other cells.

An example of adipose tissue in other organs includes epicardial adipose tissue (EAT). EAT has a role in the heart acting as a buffering system against toxic levels of fatty acids. It is thought that EAT might be a scavenger for excess fatty acids. Keeping in mind there is no structure separating adipose and myocardial layers and they share the same blood supply, it is interesting to note adiponectin has profound anti-inflammatory and antiatherogenic properties. Thus, EAT in normal amounts is likely protective to the heart.

Lipoprotein lipase is secreted by adipocytes and provides for lipids to be taken up from the circulation by breaking down triglycerides into cholesterol and fatty acids. The fatty acids are then repackaged into triglycerides for storage in the adipocyte. When the body has a need for energy, as mentioned previously, the sympathetic nervous system activates hormone-sensitive lipase which creates the release and sends fatty acids back into the circulation.

In addition to releasing fatty acids, the hormones that regulate the anorexogenic pathway increase energy expenditure by increasing basal metabolism rate. There is also an increase in spontaneous non-exercise activity thermogenesis (NEAT) such as fidgeting, pacing, and changing posture.

Leptin is one of the hormones that increase the sympathetic nervous system signaling to increase basal metabolism rate. Glucose also helps with anorexic signaling as it tells the body that there is energy available. Insulin is a powerful hormone in the hunger satiety feedback mechanism. First it reinforces glucose messaging by decreasing NPY and GRP. Insulin also increases leptin secretion. Leptin increases energy expenditure by causing a rise in T3 thereby increasing the metabolic rate. Of course, this only works if there's no leptin resistance, which is found in most patients with obesity.

There are other mediators in the energy homeostasis system. Serotonin, as we know, is involved in sleep, pain sensitivity, blood pressure, and mood regulation. It also influences energy homeostasis. It does this centrally through the hypothalamus. In the hypothalamus serotonin activates POMC neurons to reduce feeding behavior. Serotonin has been strongly linked with carbohydrate craving.

Future Use of Adipose Cells

Adipose tissue can be obtained through liposuction. In fact, there are therapeutic possibilities for the future using adipose cells as a cell-based therapy. They are stem cell tissue and show a possibility of creating bone, cartilage, and muscle and neuronal cells. *Who knew?*

Hormones

We will discuss pathophysiology in another chapter, but let's look more intensely at the hormones related to hunger, satiety, and homeostasis of weight control and a bit about what happens to them in the environment of the disease of obesity. There are many hormones involved, but our current knowledge when it comes to hunger and satiety is that the homeostatic balance uses one hunger hormone (ghrelin) and numerous hormones for satiety with leptin leading the pack.

Leptin is the hormone that tells us we are full, while ghrelin tells us we are hungry. Like most hormones they should be balancing to keep the body in homeostasis. Other hormones impact this system of the brain, stomach, intestines, and pancreas conversation. As we once thought diabetes was only about insulin and glucose, we have come a long way from that paradigm. Understanding obesity is now the same. Obesity is a disease with the homeostatic system broken.

Leptin

Leptin was the first adipokine discovered. It plays a role in food intake control, body weight control, and maintenance of energy homeostasis—its discovery showed that adipose tissue was beyond a storage site and instead an active endocrine tissue. Adipocytes are the major source of leptin.

Leptin is the signaling molecule between peripheral organs and CNS (see Fig. 3.3). Leptin has been thoroughly researched since being found in 1994. It has a role in carbohydrate, bone, and reproductive metabolism, but the greatest interest around obesity is body weight regulation. Leptins' major role in body

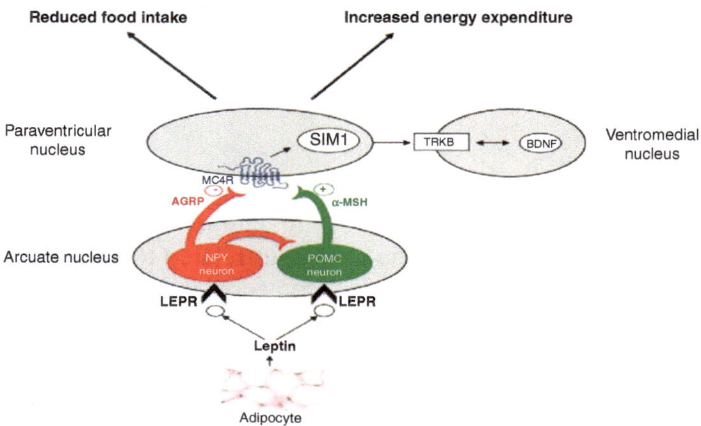

FIGURE 3.3 Leptin association to CNS

weight regulation is to signal the hypothalamus about satiety. In patients without obesity this inhibits food intake and reduces fat storage, but it also plays a role in energy expenditure and carbohydrate metabolism through the SNS. Thus leptin signals go to the hypothalamus to regulate eating behavior as well as metabolic homeostasis. The impact on energy is to increase thyrotropin releasing hormone.

Insulin increases leptin production, albeit indirectly, to allow glucose utilization in adipocytes. Conversely leptin has a direct effect on insulin secretion. There are leptin receptors in the pancreatic B cells. Its endocrine function includes decreasing insulin secretion from the B cells and insulin biosynthesis by reducing proinsulin mRNA.

Leptin can also be expressed in the ovary and placenta and by the fetus. It has a role in controlling the growth and maturation of ovarian follicles and acts as a proliferative factor. Leptin also acts as part of signaling initiating onset of puberty. Leptin may act as a growth factor for a fetus serving as a messenger controlling energy between mother and fetus.

Leptin modulates the function of the HPA axis and the systemic sympathetic/adrenomedullary system. Adrenal glands are naturally surrounded by adipose tissue and therefore are likely exposed to high concentrations of leptin, a very active hormone.

Let's look at how leptin is part of the endocrine system by demonstrating the endocrine feedback mechanism of homeostasis of energy and eating. When there is excess energy, leptin triggers a release of melanocortins. This in turn goes on to activate melanocortin 4 receptor (MC4R), a protein encoded by the MC4R gene. MC4R suppresses food intake and stimulates energy expenditure. At the same time leptin suppresses AgRP/NPY which are suppressors of MC4R.

Leptin plays a role in reward and motivation. It does this by acting on dopaminergic neurons in the ventral tegmental area (a region of the brain involved in reward and motivation) to influence eating behavior. In obesity the ability of leptin to decrease food intake is impaired due to a central leptin resistance.

Insulin

We all know insulin's role in the pancreas and glucose regulation. Only the role in food and homeostasis will be covered here. Insulin has a CNS role in controlling food intake. It is fascinating as it is catabolic in the central system while peripherally anabolic. And the central effects are mediated largely through the arcuate nucleus of the hypothalamus. The primary role of insulin is to control the levels of circulating glucose by sequestering glucose into cells after a meal and ingestion. In adipose tissue insulin promotes the uptake of fatty acids and the conversion to store triglycerides. This promotes a buildup of stored energy. Obesity is known to primarily cause insulin resistance (likely due to proinflammatory aspect of obesity). In patients with visceral adiposity higher concentrations of basal insulin are found, and there is a higher secretion of insulin in response to a standard meal.

Because insulin can cross the blood-brain barrier but is not needed by the CNS to use glucose, it is considered an adiposity signal. It functions as a hormone messenger regarding nutrition and stored fat.

Let's look at what happens with insulin in obesity. A change in insulin clearance in the liver occurs likely due to the increased concentration of free fatty acids from adipose tissue. There's also a change in the way cholesterol is metabolized (see Fig. 3.4).

CCK

Cholecystokinin is found in intestinal endocrine cells and neurons. It regulates gastric acid secretion, gastric emptying, gallbladder contraction, and exocrine pancreatic secretion. CCK may play a role in satiation through stimulation of vagal receptors signaling the hindbrain. CCK is considered a brain/gut peptide. CCK appears to be important in the communication of food intake specifically at individual meals.

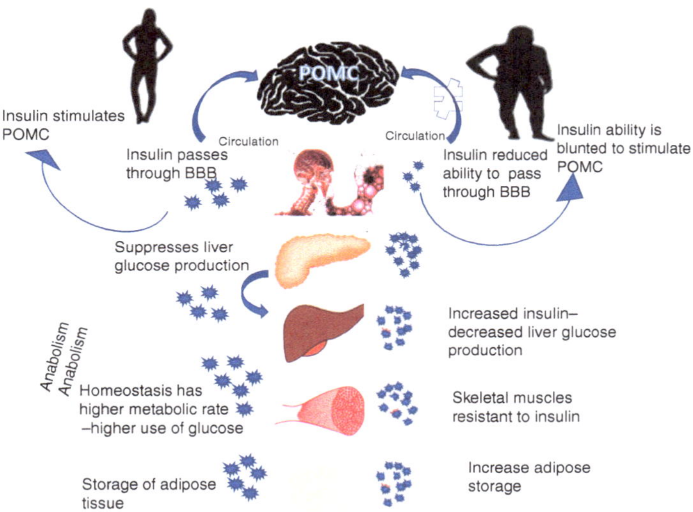

FIGURE 3.4 Insulin response in homeostasis and obesity

Adiponectin/Resistin

Adiponectin is primarily in the adipose tissue with receptors in the liver and muscle. In the liver adiponectin helps regulate insulin sensitivity and oxidation of fatty acids. It also suppresses hepatic glucose production. This hormone also stimulates thermogenesis impacting weight homeostasis. It is a powerful anti-inflammatory agent and has antifibrotic actions in the liver.

Ghrelin

Ghrelin is the only known circulating hormone with strong orexigenic activity. Ghrelin is known as the hunger hormone. Ghrelin is produced by the stomach and is a signal for eating. Its receptors are widespread almost everywhere in the body,

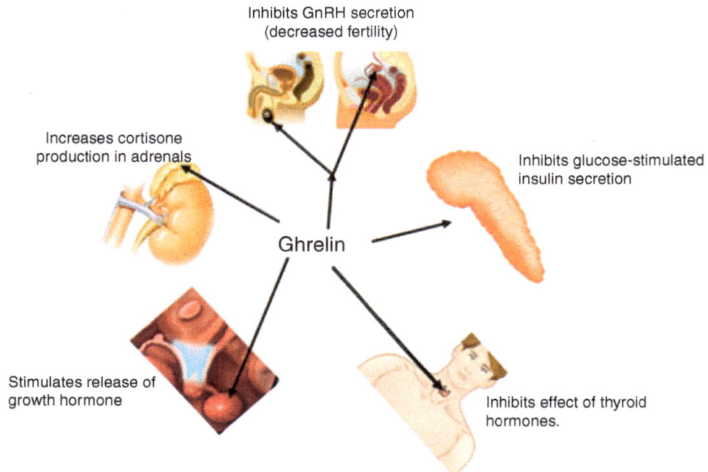

FIGURE 3.5 Ghrelin impact

but specifically in the hypothalamus and many endocrine organs including pituitary, thyroid, parathyroid, pancreas, adrenal glands, placenta, and male and female gonads (Fig. 3.5). Ghrelin is also expressed by other cells including the endocrine organs with receptors in the heart and spleen. It has also been seen in cancer cells. We have known for years about beta cells and insulin and delta cells with somatostatin, and now we see epsilon cells in the pancreas producing ghrelin.

Ghrelin crosses the blood-brain barrier and impacts the arcuate nucleus in the hypothalamus as well as the hippocampus, dorsal nucleus of the raphe, ventral tegmental area, nucleus accumbens, amygdala, prefrontal cortex nucleus, and the olfactory bulb in the control of feeding. Due to all these it is clear ghrelin regulates multiple aspects of eating including food reward, stress-induced feeding, motivation, and learning and memory responses associated with eating. Ghrelin also increases the sniffing intensity and even the willingness to spend more money on food suggesting that ghrelin increases the perceived value of food.

GLP-1

GLP-1 is produced in the small intestine and a small set of neurons in the hindbrain and inhibits eating. Endogenous GLP-1 has a very short biologic half-life. Enhanced GLP-1 release likely contributes to the anti-obesity and antidiabetic effects of bariatric surgery. Dietary carbohydrates and fat consumption simulate peripheral GLP-1 secretion. GLP-1 has been identified on the sweet receptor cells in the oral cavity suggesting that GLP-1 signaling might also be involved in taste perception. The GLP-1 receptors are widely distributed peripherally in the pancreatic islets and the entire GI tract. Centrally GLP-1 receptors are found in hypothalamus, amygdala, and in mesolimbic reward system allowing for the control of food intake and the regulation of energy balance.

Summary

As can be seen by reading this chapter, eating and energy homeostasis are incredibly complex. Adipose tissue is a metabolically active endocrine organ when in normal quantities. Additional hormones and peptides do play a role in hunger and energy in this complex system of homeostasis (Table 3.2).

Practice Pearls

- Adipose tissue has many roles beyond lipid storage and vital organ protection.
- These cells are endocrine in nature producing proteins, cytokines, and hormones.
- This is the only organ capable of continued growth throughout our life.
- Hormones and peptides must be in harmony to control appetite and energy regulation effectively.

TABLE 3.2 Additional hormones and peptides

Additional hormones impacting hunger and homeostasis of energy	
ASP	Stimulates glucose uptake, inhibits lipase, increases efficiency of triglyceride storage and synthesis
AMYLIN	Plays a role in both acute satiation and long-term control of eating. The effect of amylin is centrally mediated in the hindbrain
Peptides impacting hunger and homeostasis of energy	
Peptides—Peptides are derived from CART and POMC and are expressed in central and peripheral neurons that work on eating behaviors	CART is coexpressed with POMC in arcuate nucleus and is linked to satiety. These are stimulated by leptin
CART—cocaine- and amphetamine-regulated transcript	Occurs with food consumption, inhibits food intake, role in reward mechanism of food
POMC—proopiomelanocortin	Precursor to melanocortin. Occurs with food consumption, inhibits food intake, role in reward mechanism of food
OREXINS	Impact satiety through the vagal receptors Have been found in the intestines, pancreas, adrenal glands, reproductive system, and adipose tissue Found in many endocrine tissues including pituitary, thyroid, parathyroid, adrenals, testes, ovaries, and the pancreatic islets. Central orexins are found originating in the medulla with an impact on the HPA and affecting the SNS Impact hypothalamus for sleep and energy homeostasis beyond the impact on eating

TABLE 3.2 (continued)

Neuropeptide Y (NPY)	Found in the brain Strong control of eating in the hypothalamus encouraging an increase in food intake while decreasing energy expenditure by reducing thermogenesis Also a mediator for food rewards
Peptide YY (PYY)	Secreted by the distal gut in response to a protein rich meal. Slows gastric emptying and reduces secretions from the pancreas and gallbladder Satiety peptide In obesity PYY secretion is blunted creating a reduced feeling of satiety
Adrenomedullin	Expressed in gastrointestinal tissues including liver, pancreas, stomach, duodenum, small intestines, colon, and pancreas. Inhibits gastric and intestinal emptying Stabilizes the gut barrier Satiety

References

1. Murray S, Tulloch A, Gold MS, Avena NM. Hormonal and neural mechanisms of food reward, eating behaviour and obesity. Nat Rev Endocrinol. 2014;10(9):540–52.
2. Dietrich M, Horvath T. Limitations in anti-obesity drug development: the critical role of hunger-promoting neurons. Nat Rev Drug Discov. 2012;11(9):675–91.
3. Boulange CL, Neves AL, Chillous J, Nicholson JK, Dumas M. Impact of the gut microbiota on inflammation, obesity, and metabolic disease. Genome Med. 2016;8(42):1–12. https://doi.org/10.1186/s13073-016-0303-2.

Chapter 4
Pathophysiology of Obesity

THE JOURNEY OF 1000 MILES MUST BEGIN WITH A SINGLE STEP.

LAOZI

Introduction

This chapter examines the pathophysiology of obesity. Primarily it is the increased amount of adiposity and the defense of the increased adiposity. The dysregulation of energy homeostasis is reviewed as well as the concept of obesity as both a brain and an endocrine disease. The role of inflammation, endocrine-disrupting chemicals, and microbiome in impacting obesity is discussed. An examination of the pathologic basis of weight regain adds to the understanding of obesity as a disease.

Key Reason
In order to recognize obesity as a disease an understanding of the pathophysiology of the disease must be clearly defined. This chapter is an overview of the pathophysiology as we know it today. Much is still being learned about obesity and the pathophysiology and thereby how we, as healthcare providers, can impact the treatment is in an ever-learning state at this

A. Golden, *Treating Obesity in Primary Care*,
https://doi.org/10.1007/978-3-030-48683-9_4

time. There is a lot of information here but at the end a chart will demonstrate how the treatment of obesity can impact the pathophysiology related to the endocrine dysfunction.

There are many professional organizations that discuss the root causes of obesity. The common threads are the disease is multifactorial. We will discuss several here in this chapter. This is just an overview as there are many articles and books written about the pathophysiology of obesity. Before going any further please know I am not saying eating isn't a factor. Eating patterns and overeating are *part* of the cause of obesity—but only part. There are genetic, physiologic, environmental, and behavioral influences. Some experts like Dr. Nikhil Dhurandhar, past president of The Obesity Society and William Hardy Endowed Chair in Obesity Research, suggested (August 2018) "…eventually we will identify many different types of obesity. So let's move forward to debunk the myth of 'eat less, move more' and learn to treat obesity."

Adiposity and Defense of Increased Adiposity

There are two separate yet interconnected processes that are at the core of obesity:

1. Increase in amount of adiposity
2. Biological defense of the increased adiposity

The first point has a complex cause with genetics, environment, and biology intertwining. A defense of the increased level of adiposity occurs in obesity. Because of this eating less for short periods of time does not seem to be sufficient in the majority of patients to treat obesity.

There is good evidence of many variables that can impact our energy balance. A short list includes sleep deprivation, decreased changes in environmental temperature (thanks to heating and air conditioning), prescribed medications that cause weight gain, intranatal exposure to lack of nutrition or maternal obesity, and patients who stop smoking.

The brain and body prefer homeostasis, so when we reduce our energy intake (eat less), physiologic mechanisms such as the central orexigenic signal to increase appetite. We know that obesity or excess adiposity evolves slowly over time. Dr. Bray is one of the original researchers of obesity and recognized its pathophysiology in the early 1960s with often cited works. Recently he wrote, “Growing evidence suggests that obesity is a disorder of the energy homeostasis system” [1] (p, 267). This is greater than calories as a passive accumulation of excess weight with obesity. The body has a dysregulation in energy homeostasis defending a higher level of adipose tissue. How this happens is the subject of a lot of research for a full answer. But it has been shown that people without obesity or the propensity for obesity when overfed do not have a sustained weight gain [2]. Although recent research links genetic and environment factors as the cause of obesity, the pathophysiology is a dysfunction of the adipose tissue.

The body can only use food in two ways; it can use it for fuel or it can store it in adipose cells. When the balance of energy expenditure and energy intake becomes out of sync, the body stores the excess intake in adipose cells.

Adipocyte tissue can increase through hypertrophy or hyperplasia (the number of adipocyte cells). With hypertrophy there’s greater storage of triglycerides within each cell. It appears that hypertrophy occurs first, and when an area has become saturated with triglycerides, then hyperplasia occurs (adipocytes enlarge and then cleave into two cells). More cells mean more capacity for lipid storage. The larger the adipocyte, the less responsive to insulin, and we start to see an increase in local and systemic inflammatory responses. This inflammatory response increases the risk for insulin resistance, NASH, as well as coronary artery disease to name a few. When the multiplication of adipocytes occurs, we start to see ectopic fat deposition. This occurs in the liver, muscles, kidneys, and heart [3].

As adipocytes remodel and enlarge, there is an increase in macrophages and other immune cells. The immune cells secrete cytokines that add to the underlying cause of the

Table 4.1 Proinflammation of adipocytes

Proinflammatory secretions of adipocytes	Tumor necrosis factor alpha Interleukin-6 Monocyte chemoattractant protein-1 Lipotransin Plasminogen activator inhibitor II
Increase specifically for cardiovascular risk	Adipocyte lipid-binding protein Acylstimulation protein Prostaglandins

inflammation. Sick adipose tissue also secretes inflammatory factors (see Table 4.1). This inflammation contributes to the insulin resistance seen in most patients with obesity.

For most patients with obesity, their increase in adiposity was slow over many years. This sustained, yet incremental increase in body fat mass for an unknown reason due to the interlinking of genetics, environment, and biology becomes the energy homeostasis new point [1].

Brain Disease

The arcuate nucleus in the hypothalamus uses neuropeptides to control energy balance. This balance is central and peripheral (Fig. 4.1).

Some experts, like Dr. Hamdy, Director of the Obesity Clinic at the Joslin Diabetes Center, and Dr. Sicat, American Board of Obesity Medicine Diplomate (May 2018), talk about obesity as a brain disease. In their presentations they discuss stress-related chronic stimulation of the hypothalamic–pituitary–adrenal axis and increased glucocorticoid exposure as an important pathophysiologic factor in the development of obesity. Patients with obesity have lower levels of natriuretic peptides. The natriuretic peptides mediate endocrine and behavioral response to stress. Peripheral natri-

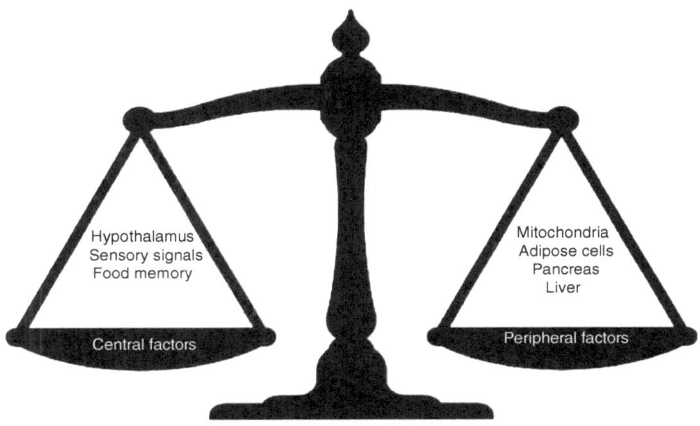

FIGURE 4.1 Scale of central and peripheral factors

uretic peptides could lead to decreased lipolysis and energy expenditure playing a role in excessive weight gain.

Endocrine Disease

The Endocrine Society and the American Association of Clinical Endocrinologist explain obesity as an endocrine disorder looking at the metabolic dysfunction. This includes over- or underproduction of adipokines and cytokines, impairments in hormonal conversion, or the body's response to hormones.

Infectious Etiology

Adenovirus-36 (AD36) was shown to be associated with obesity in chickens and mice [4]. When looking at humans however, only 20–30% have shown an infection with adenovirus-36. The study also showed higher antibody titers for AD36 in patients with obesity compared to people without obesity. This may be a cause for some but is unlikely to be a cause for every patient with obesity [4]. This provides some evidence of possible infectious etiology in the mix of the variance of obesity. Of equal interest is that this infection is only seen in 5% of people who do not have obesity [5].

Genetic Factor

Phenotypes of obesity make this a complex disease to determine best treatment for an individual patient. The Endocrine Society summarizes genetic influence as a contribution to the disease. In a study of the genetic basis of obesity complications, they were able to demonstrate that weight loss can cause a modification in the expression of over 100 genes. The study showed not just the link with genes but what could happen with treatment [6]. It is likely an interaction of the risk alleles with the environment, epigenetic factors, and influences of development. GWAS data has shown us there is no one gene causing obesity except in very rare situations. Dr. Michelle Look, a board-certified obesity specialist and the team physician for USA Rugby, says instead "genetics is the lock and the environment is the key" (March 16, 2019). In other words, genetics isn't the cause but creates a susceptibility based on environmental influences.

The FTO gene encodes fat mass and obesity-associated protein and is thought to impact the amount of fat mass a person is *capable* of having. In large studies of the genome, there have been over 300 loci identified, but this is likely not the majority of the cases of obesity. The real cause of obesity may be more about how the environment is making epigenomic changes to the DNA. These genetic variants are likely where we see the susceptibility to obesity [7]. These epigenomic changes occur without the actual modification of the DNA sequencing. Many experts believe this may be the real cause of the individual differences in the phenotypes of obesity traits [8]. There are rare forms of monogenic forms of obesity. The most common of the rare forms of obesity causes severe disease in children due to melanocortin 4 receptor gene deficit.

Inflammation

The pathophysiology related to chronic low-level inflammation includes the activation of the immune system with production of cytokines. This promotes the production of mast cells and macrophages. The production of cytokines, such as tumor necrosis factor α (TNF-α) or interleukin (IL)-1β, leads to impaired insulin action, aka resistance, leading to the development of metabolic abnormalities.

Endocrine-Disrupting Chemicals

Another theory related to obesity causation is the endocrine-disrupting chemicals (EDCs). The WOF epidemiologic model for obesity believes that the environment impacts on a person to produce the disease of obesity [1]. Many of the EDCs we have heard of are bisphenol A (BPA) and perfluorinated compounds (PFCs). Some have now been banned. The rise of exposure to EDCs parallels the increase of obesity rates. Studies have shown the EDCs can stimulate adipogenesis and disrupt liver metabolism and insulin sensitivity [1]. PFCs are widely used to make products more resistant to stains, grease, and water. Because they break down in the environment very slowly, they tend to accumulate and can therefore persist in human tissues for years. PFCs may impact the peroxisome proliferator–activated receptor and dysregulate adipogenesis. This is important as research is looking at PPAR as a possible treatment intervention.

BPA is part of the production of polycarbonate plastics we are exposed through bottles, food-can linings, and food packaging [9]. This may or may not be a cause of obesity but may be one of the many environmental factors that predispose a person to obesity via epigenetic changes. One observation is that EDCs could change the microbiome, allowing the gut to absorb more calories from food in patients with obesity [7].

Microbiome

There is interesting evidence of the probability that the gut bacteria from the small and large intestines are affecting energy balance by influencing the signals to the brain.

Inflammation

There is a great deal of chronic low-grade inflammation with obesity. Animal models demonstrate inflammation in the hypothalamus [10]. Perhaps this inflammation that is occurring with high fat diets in animals creates an injury that allows the increase in the body defense as obesity begins and continues. It is hypothesized that the inflammation may injure neurons and keep them from responding to leptin or other peptide signals to keep a lower fat mass defense. Could this be a cause in humans? We don't know, but it is an intriguing hypothesis that many researchers are investigating.

Behavior

Food and activity impact

- *Do consumed carbohydrates impact obesity rates?* Multiple researchers have shown that sugars increase insulin secretion. Insulin suppresses lipolysis and the release of fatty acids from adipose tissue. It also plays a role in directing dietary fat to storage. However, this doesn't play out with everyone. So, the answer is carbohydrates aren't a simple causation of obesity [11].
- *Is it all about lack of activity?*
  On the surface increased activity (aka exercise) should promote a negative balance, right? Not so fast. What we find instead is patients with obesity have a mechanism for homeostasis that promotes increased energy intake with exercise. There does seem to be an effect on energy

homeostasis that may impact keeping obesity in check when in a maintenance phase of treatment.

Smoking Cessation

Why does smoking cessation have an association with weight gain? This is most likely due to withdrawal of the pharmacological effect of nicotine. Nicotine suppresses food intake. The mechanism for this is in the hypothalamus where POMC neurons are activated through nicotinic acetylcholine receptors that reduce food intake [12]. This is not a recommendation to smoke! We all know how severe the long-term impact is on our bodies with smoking. It is just an explanation for how smoking cessation can impact the disease of obesity [4].

Weight Regain

Over time most patients who have successfully lost weight find that they regain the weight and sometimes a bit more. Most patients will express how they have been unsuccessful at weight loss. This is not actually true. Almost every patient with obesity has had 7–10 concerted attempts at weight loss but have not been able to maintain the weight loss. Rather than viewing recovery of lost weight as a therapeutic failure or evidence of noncompliance, patients and providers need to view this as an expected physiological response to weight loss, now being referred to as metabolic adaptation [13].

After weight loss, many feel increased hunger. Increased appetite and decreased satiety after weight loss are associated with an increase in the 24-hour profile of circulating levels of the orexigenic hormone ghrelin and reductions in the levels of the anorexigenic hormones PYY, CCK, leptin, and insulin. These adaptive changes, associated with appetite-related hormones, appear to persist for at least 1 year after weight reduction and may remain altered indefinitely, promoting increased energy intake and ultimately weight regain.

Thus, long-term strategies are needed to prevent obesity relapse and sustain weight loss [14].

There are two pathways to consider when looking at the body's capability of maintaining a steady weight. The first path is orexigenic, or appetite stimulating, and the second path is anorexigenic, or appetite suppressing [3]. These pathways are mediated through the neuroendocrine signal system. The adipocytes, gut-derived signals, and skeletal muscle performance are all part of the communication. Excluding what might be happening in bariatric surgery, the primary treatment of obesity continues to rely on creating a negative energy balance. There is no consistent definition of weight regain after weight loss. However, in reviewing literature, it seems that successful treatment is considered 10% total body weight loss for medical management and that regain is less than 3% of their body weight. Some researchers have demonstrated that two thirds of all who've lost weight regain more weight than was lost when using only dietary intervention. Many of us have heard of the set point theory but few realize that this was created in 1972 by Nesbitt [15]. The theory says the individual weight is maintained and is a state of equilibrium between energy storage and utilization. Since for many people weight gain has occurred over years if not decades one has to wonder why the system didn't keep them at a lower weight, a.k.a. a normal weight. Fifty years later we still don't really understand the process that leads to obesity and whether or not the set point theory can be readily explained in patients with obesity.

Weight regain is likely a compensatory mechanism designed to prevent a severe catabolic state due to the following:

- Reduction in leptin secretion. With decreased leptin, there is an increase in the orexigenic peptides.
- Energy expenditure reduces by 15% over 24 hours likely due to an increase in parasympathetic system activity.
- T3 secretion declines, but it's unlikely to appear as clinical hypothyroidism.

- Alteration in hypothalamic energy signaling, and this may persist for years, even with weight regain [16].
- Skeletal muscle becomes more efficient with weight loss, thereby requiring fewer calories in order to do the work that the person was doing before weight loss.

Dr. Garvey, past president of the American Association of Clinical Endocrinologist, published on weight regain saying "…once weight has been lost our bodies are wired by the disease to regain the weight." The changes with weight loss include decreased resting metabolism rate, increased ghrelin (appetite-stimulating hormone), as well as decreased leptin (satiety hormone). This is physiology not willpower (Obesity Action Coalition, n.d.).

So What Is Metabolic Adaptation?

Metabolic adaptation is an activation of hormonal changes that create an environment for weight regain. This demonstrates the relapsing part of the disease [8]. Sumitharin [14] demonstrated that hormonal adaptation occurs after weight loss at 10 weeks and 62 weeks. The hormones measured were those associated hunger and satiety, ghrelin, insulin, leptin, PYY, CCK, and GLP-1. All individuals demonstrated lower levels of satiety hormones and increased hunger hormone.

Beyond hunger and satiety metabolic adaptation is adaptive thermogenesis causing a decreasing energy expenditure. Lean body mass that is lost with dieting may be lowering the resting energy expenditure. There's evidence to support that the degree of metabolic adaptation could be independent of total baseline body fat [17].

Are There Any Benefits Even with Weight Regain?

Bluher and associates [18] demonstrated that even patients with weight regain showed long-lasting improvements in high density lipoprotein, and inflammatory markers like C reactive protein indicate that patients benefit even after weight regain from their weight loss.

Clinical Practice Implication

What does all this mean for clinical practice. Looking at the pathophysiology makes one wonder if medical management treatment can be successful. The beliefs of society, and in fact most of healthcare, are that treating obesity is simply eating less and moving more. Decades have clearly demonstrated this is a poor paradigm and instead we must recognize that the body's energy balance and adiposity are controlled by biologic processes that are resistant to the usual treatment of changing calories and activity. We must look beyond diet and exercise for the treatment of the chronic and lifelong disease of obesity (see Table 4.2). We should also look beyond the number on the scale for other measurement: improved sleep patterns, benefits of physical activity for the complications of obesity, and improving metabolic markers.

Table 4.2 What can be done about the hormones of appetite

Intervention	Hormone/organ	Process
Physical activity	Insulin	Allows us to burn those glycogen stores [19] 10-minute walks in people with diabetes immediately after a meal decreased the postprandial glucose and dinner was most impactful with a 27% decrease
Sleep	Leptin	Decreases with too little sleep
Exercise	Leptin	Increases leptin sensitivity
Avoid processed food	Integrity of gut	Decreases inflammation

TABLE 4.2 (continued)

Intervention	Hormone/organ	Process
Eat soluble fiber	Integrity of gut	Improves your gut health and may protect against obesity
Reduced carbohydrate intake	Triglycerides	Lowers triglycerides to prevent the transport of leptin from our blood to brain
Eat protein	Leptin	Improvement in leptin sensitivity
Decreased carbohydrates, increase protein and fiber	Ghrelin	Increases the stretch of stomach to increase satiety
Low carbohydrate, increase protein and fiber	Peptide YY	Increases satiety
Sleep, activity, and stress management	Cortisol	Decreased cortisol decreases appetite
Meal that is a combination of protein, fiber, and healthy fats	Cholecystokinin	Slows gastric emptying and decreasing meal volume
Protein and polyphenols (leafy greens)	GLP-1	Increases GLP-1
Stress management	NYP	Increases NYP and satiety

Conclusion

The pathologic basis of obesity is excess adipose tissue. The sequela of this is that adipose cells enlarge to capacity and then there is an increase in deposition of adipose in organs like the liver, heart, kidney, and muscle. Added to this is the interaction of the adipose cell and the microbiome with an increase in inflammation. As the adipose mass increases and becomes pathologic, it produces peptides, cytokines, and free fatty acids while decreasing the production of adiponectin. All these changes seem to be occurring due to a genetic predisposition or epigenetic changes that are impacted by the obesogenic environment we live in.

Practice Pearls

- Obesity is a complex disease with the increase in cytokines and decrease in adiponectin.
- Inflammation likely plays a role in the increase fat mass and defense of the fat mass.
- Obesity has different causes for different people and is not one disease.
- Weight regain is a physiologic process *not* lack of willpower.

References

1. Bray GA, Kim KK, Wilding JPH, World Obesity Federation. Obesity: a chronic relapsing progressive disease process. A position statement of the World Obesity Federation. Obes Rev. 2017;18(7):715–23.
2. Leibel RL, Rosenbaum M, Hirsch J. Changes in energy expenditure resulting from altered body weight. N Engl J Med. 1995;332:621–8.
3. Rogge M, Gautam B. Biology of obesity and weight regain: implications for clinical practice. J Am Assoc Nurse Pract. 2017;29:S15–29.
4. Dhurandhar N, Bailey D, Thomas D. Interaction of obesity and infections. Obes Rev. 2015;16:1017–29.
5. Ponterio E, Gnessi L. Adenovirus 36 and obesity: an overview. Viruses. 2015;7:3719–40.
6. Skrypnik K, Suliburska J, Skrypnik D, Pilarski T, Reguta J, Bogdanski P. The genetic basis of obesity complications. Acta Sci Pol Technol. 2017;16(1):83–91.
7. Boulange CL, Neves AL, Chillous J, Nicholson JK, Dumas M. Impact of the gut microbiota on inflammation, obesity, and metabolic disease. Genome Med. 2016;8:42):1–12. https://doi.org/10.1186/s13073-016-0303-2.

8. Heymsfield SB, Wadden TA. Mechanisms, pathophysiology and management of obesity. N Engl J Med. 2017;376(3):254–66.
9. Chapin R, Adams J, Boekelheide K, Gray L, Hayward S, Lees P, et al. NTP-CERHR expert panel report on the reproductive and developmental toxicity of bisphenol A. Birth Defects Res B Dev Reprod Toxicol. 2008;83:157–395.
10. Valdearcos M, Robblee MM, Benjamin DI, Nomura DK, Xu AW, Kowliwad SK. Microglia dictate the impact of saturated fat consumption on hypothalamic inflammation and neuronal function. Cell Rep. 2014;9(6):2124–38.
11. Knowler W, Fowler S, Hamman R, Christophi C, Hoffman H, Diabetes Prevention Program Research Group, et al. 10-year follow-up of diabetes incidence and weight loss in the Diabetes Prevention Program Outcomes Study. Lancet. 2009;374(9702):1677–86.
12. Mineur S, Abizaid A, Rao Y, Salas R, DiLeone R, Gundisch D, et al. Nicotine decreases food intake through activation of POMC neurons. Science. 2011;332:1330–2.
13. Kaplan LM, Golden A, Jinnett K, Kolotkin RL, Kyle TK, Look M, et al. Perceptions of barriers to effective obesity care: results from the national ACTION study. Obesity. 2016;26:61. https://doi.org/10.1002/oby.22054.
14. Sumithran P, Prendergast LA, Delbridge E, Purcell K, Shulkes A, Kriketos A, Proietto J. Long-term persistence of hormonal adaptations to weight loss. N Engl J Med. 2001;365(17):1597–604.
15. Nisbett RE. Hunger, obesity, and the ventromedial hypothalamus. Psychol Rev. 1972;79:433–53.
16. Maclean PS, Bergouignan A, Cornier MA, Jackman MR. Biology's response to dieting: the impetus for weight regain. Am J Physiol Regul Integr Comp Physiol. 2011;301(3):R581–600. https://doi.org/10.1152/ajpregu.00755.2010.
17. Howell S, Kones R. "Calories in, calories out" and macronutrient intake: the hope, hype, and science of calories. Am J Physiol Endocrinol Metab. 2017;313:E608–12.
18. Bluher M, Rudich A, Kloting N, Golan R, Henkin Y, Rubin E, et al. Two patterns of adipoline and other biomarker dynamics in a long-term weight loss intervention. Diabetes Care. 2012;35(2):342–9. and associates.
19. Reynolds AN, Mann JI, Williams S, Venn BJ. Advice to walk after meals is more effective for lowering postprandial glycaemia in type 2 diabetes mellitus than advice that does not specify timing: a randomized crossover study. Diabetologia. 2016;59:2572–8.

Chapter 5
Obesity-Related Complications

> *IT AIN'T WHAT YOU KNOW THAT GET YOU IN TROUBLE,*
>
> *IT'S WHAT YOU KNOW FOR SURE BUT JUST AIN'T SO.*
>
> *MARK TWAIN*

Key Reason
Obesity is recognized as a chronic disease partially because it has identified complications. This is the basis of the rationale of why obesity must be treated. By treating obesity so many other diseases are being impacted at the same time thus treating the root cause of some diseases versus just the symptoms. This chapter will look at some of the complications and the pathophysiology that explain the underlying issues. More importantly the chapter explains why it matters for the clinical implications.

Introduction

This chapter examines how the complications of obesity are part of defining obesity as a disease (Table 5.1). A review of

A. Golden, *Treating Obesity in Primary Care*,
https://doi.org/10.1007/978-3-030-48683-9_5

Table 5.1 Obesity-related complications: disorders or diseases with obesity as a cause

System	Disease
Respiratory	Increased respiratory infections Increased incidence and severity of asthma Pickwickian syndrome
Immunologic	Increase in incidence of cancer: endometrial (premenopausal), prostate, colon, post-menopausal breast cancer, gallbladder, gastric, pancreatic, ovarian, and renal to list a few
Cardiovascular	Coronary heart disease Essential hypertension Left ventricular hypertrophy Cor pulmonale Cardiomyopathy Accelerated atherosclerosis Pulmonary hypertension of obesity Atrial fibrillation Varicosities Lymphedema
Central nervous system	TIA and CVA Idiopathic intracranial hypertension Meralgia paresthetica
Obstetric and perinatal	Pregnancy related HTN Fetal macrosomia Pelvic dystocia Stress incontinence Anovulation Early puberty Infertility Hyperandrogenism POCS Stress incontinence
Reproductive: men	Hypogonadotropic hypogonadism
GI	Cholecystitis, cholelithiasis NAFLD, steatohepatitis GERD

Table 5.1 (continued)

System	Disease
Orthopedics	Osteoarthritis Slipped capital femoral epiphyses Blount disease Legg-Calve-Perthes disease Chronic low back pain
Metabolic	Per-diabetes, T2DM Metabolic syndrome Dyslipidemia
Cutaneous	Intertrigo Acanthosis nigricans Increased risk of cellulitis and carbuncles Hirsutism
Renal	Increase in kidney stones Fatty kidney disease
Obesity-related comorbidities: disorders or diseases that impact obesity and obesity can worsen	
Respiratory	Obstructive sleep
Psychologic	Depression Anxiety Stigmatization

Multiple references were used for the chart, and it by no means covers all the ORCs but gives an overview of complications [1–3]

several of the complications and the pathophysiology of obesity causes the complications. An assessment of the clinical implications is discussed.

AACE [4] proposed an advanced framework for a patient with a diagnosis of obesity. This document demonstrates adipose tissue as an endocrine organ which can become dysfunctional and contribute to systematic metabolic disease. Based on this view treatment of obesity is then used to prevent or treat metabolic disease by improving adipose tissue function. Zheng [5] analyzed data of US women from the Nurses' Health Study and US men from Health Professionals

Follow-Up Study and found that these health professionals had an increase in major chronic disease and less chance of healthy aging if they gained weight during adult years.

Let's look at the seminal study of obesity-associated disorders (OAD). Yeun and colleagues [1] presented the findings at Obesity Week 2016. The study reviewed literature to evaluate the extent of OADs. Their primary aim was to assess the relationship between the severity of obesity and the risk of having an OAD. They used BMI and waist circumference as the measurements for determinants in their literature search. About 236 OADs were identified in the presentation. The OADs are identified with circle size and color. The size of the circles related to the number of articles found while the color indicated the graded strength of association (see Fig. 5.1). As an example, the findings demonstrated 50 obesity-associated disorders related to women's health and 16 obesity-associated cancers.

All-Cause Mortality

Obesity identified as Stage 2 (ACEE staging) or Stage 2–4 (EOSS staging) is associated with significantly higher all-cause mortality. We do not yet have studies to understand if a patient with preobesity (overweight) or a patient with a lower BMI and less severe complications may have an increase in morbidity and mortality; however, it is clear that preventing worsening of the disease is imperative.

Cancer

The cancer progress report from the American Association for Cancer Research [6] reported that in 2014 obesity-related cancer comprised 40% of all the cancer cases in the USA. Consider the rise in the disease of obesity since 2014 (37%) to 2018 (39%) adding 5 million more adults with obesity and it is easy to see how obesity can affect public

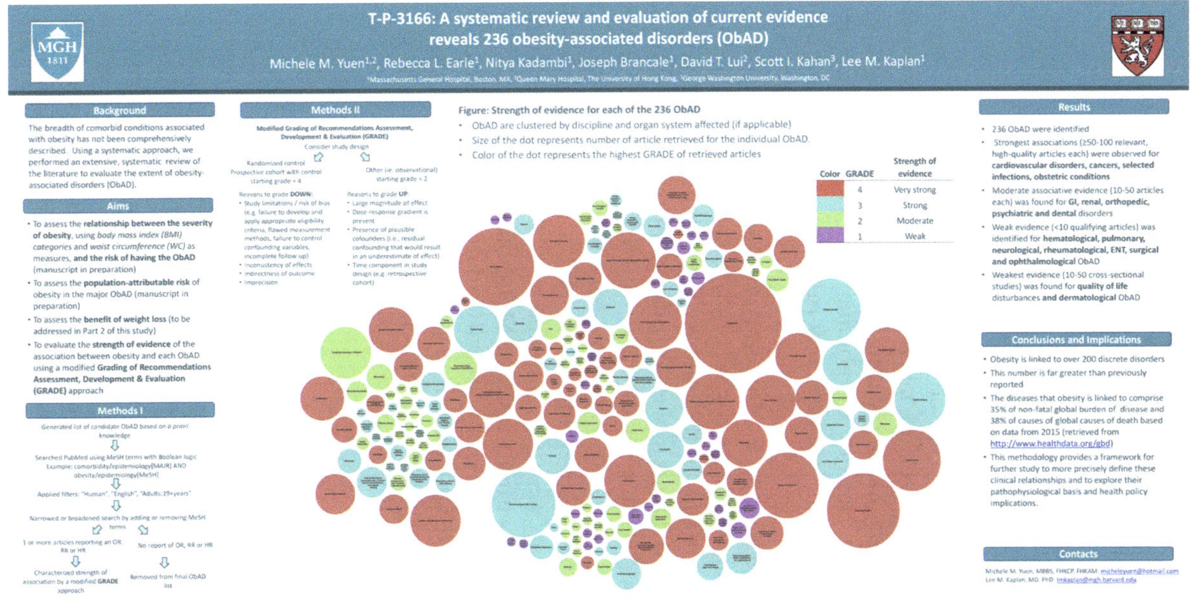

FIGURE 5.1 Review of obesity-associated disorders

health. Obesity ranks as second only to tobacco use for cancer risk. Additionally, patients with obesity have more aggressive forms of cancer and are diagnosed at a more advanced disease stage.

Mechanism

Excess adipose tissue produces hormones like estrogen and increased levels of insulin and insulin-like growth factor 1. These are likely creating an environment for the development of cancers. Combining this with increased levels of leptin which promotes cell proliferation and more rapid cell division, these are likely factors in tumor cell aggression.

When adipose tissue has outgrown adequate vascular supply, macrophages arrive to do cleanup, but in so doing they summon their inflammatory friends through cytokine signaling. This equals low-grade inflammation which is also thought to be a factor for cancers overall [7]. A longer duration of overweight and obesity is associated with increased risk of developing several forms of cancer [8]. This is likely the reason that we find patients with later disease than those patients without obesity. Metabolic dysregulation has been identified as a risk of obesity-related cancers. Parekh [7] demonstrated that increased impaired fasting glucose increases the risk of obesity-related cancers particularly colorectal cancer.

Clinical Implications

Women with preexisting obesity-related complications and any weight loss had a 20% reduction in all-cause mortality primarily due to reduced mortality from cancers and diabetes [3]. Reducing impaired fasting glucose and decreasing inflammation can reduce the cancers that confront patients. Our impact in cancer incidence and outcome is a great reason to assertively treat obesity. Reducing inflammation can reduce cancer. We need to be especially vigilant with cancer screening for our patients with obesity. So many of our patients aren't getting this as they avoid healthcare.

Liver

Nonalcoholic fatty liver disease (NAFLD) affects 60–80% of patients with DM and obesity and 100% of people with severe obesity. It parallels the obesity epidemic in the USA and is now the most common hepatic disease in the Western Hemisphere [9]. Currently it is the third leading indication for transplant, but it is estimated by 2030 nonalcoholic steatosis hepatitis is predicted to become the most common reason for transplant in the USA [10].

Mechanisms

NAFLD is a manifestation of pathologic ectopic fat in the liver combined with a low-grade chronic inflammatory state. The liver is an organ that does not work well with accumulated adipose tissue. The hepatocytes become vulnerable to lipid oxidation, impaired apoptosis, and cytokine activity. Let's take a step back and review the pathophysiology of excess adipose tissue. Adipose tissue produces free fatty acids and adipokines. This then increases TNF-α, resistin, and interleukin 6. There's also a decrease in adiponectin and an increase in insulin resistance. All this increases ectopic fat accumulation and inflammation, including in the liver. When excess adiposity occurs in the liver, liposomes, which are small organelles near mitochondria, increase in size. This creates steatosis, further leading to nonalcoholic fatty liver disease, steatohepatitis, and even cirrhosis [2]. Adiponectin promotes the synthesis of HDL cholesterol, but with obesity there are lower levels of adiponectin which is likely the underlying mechanism of lipid abnormalities associated with obesity.

Clinical Implications

The clinical implications R/T NALFD is that the treatment starts with treating obesity. Seven percent weight loss from baseline gives significant improvements in steatosis and lobular inflammation [11]. Nine percent body weight loss showed histologic improvement although this may require as much as 40% weight loss [12]. The therapeutic imperative for patients with NAFLD is to slow down or stop disease progression from hepatic steatosis to NASH to cirrhosis to liver failure and/or adenocarcinoma. Bariatric surgery literature reports some patients experience complete resolution of NASH. The anti-obesity medications recommended by AACE include orlistat and liraglutide [3].

Kidneys

ORG

We have a whole new disease thanks to obesity: obesity-related glomerulopathy (ORG). ORG is defined pathologically as glomerulomegaly and focal segmental glomerulosclerosis (FSGS) which describes scarring in the kidney that occurs in patients with a BMI $\geq$ 30 kg/m^2. ORG is a risk factor for chronic kidney disease in adults and children with the increased occurrence and faster progression, nephrolithiasis, and kidney cancer.

Mechanism

Fatty kidney is a triglyceride accumulation in the kidney. This increases GFR, RPF, filtration fraction, and tubular reabsorption of sodium promoting glomerular hypertension [13]. Beyond the fat deposit with inflammation, oxidative stress activates the renin-angiotensin-aldosterone system. Insulin resistance, characteristic of obesity, and its impacts on tubular sodium and hydrogen exchange causes additional problems. ORG criteria to diagnosis are BMI $\geq$ 30 kg/m^2 and glomerulomegaly (with or without FSGS). An initial clinical feature is isolated proteinuria. Patients with obesity and type II diabetes may create difficulty in determining whether diabetes or obesity has the prominent role in the development of proteinuria. Other common findings are hypertension (in 50–75% of patients) and dyslipidemia (in 70–80% of patients) [14]. The reasons why patients with ORG do not develop the typical findings of nephrotic syndrome, hyperlipidemia, hypoalbuminemia, and edema probably relate to the type of podocyte injury and a fairly slow development of proteinuria as well as an adaptive forms of FSGS [15].

Clinical Implications

Preventing chronic kidney disease can occur with weight loss. It is believed that the scarring of the kidney is not likely to be reversed, but further damage can be prevented.

Chronic Kidney Disease

Mechanism

The mechanism for ectopic fat deposit is based on patients with obesity having a compensatory hyperfiltration that occurs to meet the heightened metabolic demands of the increased bodyweight. The increase in intraglomerular pressure can damage the kidneys and raise the risk of developing CKD in the long term. Studies have shown impairment of intestinal barrier function and changes in the composition of the microbiome may also contribute to the prevailing inflammation associated with CKD [15].

Clinical Mechanism

Treating obesity by reducing bodyweight has shown reductions in blood pressure, glomerular hyperfiltration, and proteinuria. Additionally, eating high fiber foods may be the main driver by which the microbiota is modified. High fiber diet promotes growth of short chain fatty acid producing bacteria in the intestines and has been demonstrated in preclinical studies to be effective in treating metabolic syndrome, obesity, and CKD. Increased fiber intake is associated with decreased inflammation and decrease in all-cause mortality in patients with CKD [15]. Bariatric surgery intervention has been suggested for selected CKD and end-stage renal disease patients including patients on dialysis who were waitlisted for kidney transplantation. Bariatric surgery–induced weight loss might preserve or improve kidney function and modifies the intestinal microbiota [15].

Medications to consider for patients with obesity and chronic kidney disease include the RAAS blockade medications; remember that the beneficial effects of RAAS blockers become exhausted overtime. SGLT-2 inhibitors may have renal protective mechanism and may help with some weight loss. In relation to anti-obesity medications, orlistat and liraglutide can be used. Caution may be appropriate with orlistat as it has had an increased risk of stones, same with phentermine/topiramate [3].

Metabolic

Mechanism

Obesity increases production of free fatty acids and adipose tissue is deposited in tissues that normally take up glucose such as muscle and liver. This leads to decreased insulin sensitivity to glucose and thereby insulin resistance. So, we get a vicious cycle of insulin resistance increased free fatty acids, increased fatty deposits, and furthering increased insulin resistance.

Prediabetes

The World Health Organization has defined prediabetes as a state of intermediate hyperglycemia [16].

Mechanism

It's possible that due to continuous exposure of non-esterified fatty acids (NEFA), a free fatty acid produced by adipose tissues, reduced insulin synthesis, and increasing resistance occurs.

Diabetes

Diabetes with obesity has been referred to as diabesity [17].

Mechanism

The pathophysiology of T2DM is decreased insulin sensitivity and eventual decrease in secretion. Obesity impacts both of these. Obesity has been shown to worsen insulin resistance and exacerbate the metabolic environment that is directly toxic to β cells, including inflammation, lipotoxicity, and glucose toxicity. Obesity causes a decrease in β-cell mass and a decreased response to the incretins which impact the ability of cells to uptake glucose. Diabetes is known to have endothelial dysfunction that is worsened by obesity. We know that in diabetes β cells can no longer compensate and therefore hyperglycemia results. Type II diabetes represents a disease arising from insulin resistance and the progression of cardiometabolic disease.

Clinical Implication

The Diabetes Prevention Program demonstrated that treating obesity decreases the risk of T2DM. For every kg of weight loss there was a 16% reduction in type II diabetes risk. The combined data from numerous studies suggest that 10% weight loss will reduce the risk of future type II diabetes by 80%.

ACCE [4] recommends orlistat, phentermine/topiramate ER, or liraglutide for patients at risk for diabetes, added to intensive lifestyle intervention in order to obtain 10% weight loss. ACEE recommends that diabetes medications would be added only if the above is unsuccessful [3]. ACEE guideline also recommends carefully utilizing antidiabetes medications that can contribute to weight loss (e.g., GLP-1, SGLT2-I, and metformin). If the above fail, they recommend bariatric surgery (Roux-en-Y, sleeve gastrectomy, or BPD).

Metabolic Syndrome

Mechanism

The pathophysiology of metabolic syndrome is that high plasma glucose and insulin resistance occur with exposure to high free fatty acid. These are a common mediator and a consequence of increased intra-abdominal fat mass.

Clinical Indications

Clinical indications are the same as insulin resistance and prediabetes. The goal is to prevent or reduce diabetes and cardiovascular disease. A modest weight loss of 5–10% has been shown to substantially benefit all metabolic risk factors for patients.

Cardiovascular

Cardiovascular disease has long been linked to obesity. Prior to discussing mechanisms, a quick review of two types of adipose tissue is needed. Periaortic adipose tissue (PAT) is found around the aorta and other systemic vessels, although it is not found in the brain vascular system. Epicardial adipose tissue (EAT) is located around the coronary arteries. Both of these have physiologic purposes with PAT as part of the protection of large vessels, and EAT is metabolically active form of adipose tissue that in its normal proportion is a major source of anti-inflammatory adipokines like adiponectin. Adiponectin is a peptide hormone produced only by adipose cells and has antiatherogenic, antioxidative, and anti-inflammatory properties. EAT is also responsible for release of adrenomedullin which is a potent vasodilator peptide. PAT and EAT are capable of regulating vascular tone by variation in the size of their cell diameters.

Mechanism

Obesity's connection is most likely through the low systemic inflammation that can contribute to atherosclerotic processes. Adults with obesity between the ages of 45 and 64 die 12.8 years earlier than those of normal weight [18]. When adipocytes get bigger, oxygen diffusion can be impaired and oxygen supply is reduced due to a decrease in capillary density. In a recent study obesity and high fat diet can cause increased oxygen consumption in adipocytes [19]. Oxygen shortage in adipose tissue leads to the production of adipokines and pro-inflammatory cytokines, but also to an impaired glucose homeostasis and lipid metabolism [20]. Furthermore, hypoxia also inhibits adipogenic differentiation, which favors adipocyte enlargement. Low systemic inflammation is known to be responsible for insulin resistance and contributes to atherosclerotic processes. It is important to note that obesity does not always result in vascular endothelial dysfunction, this may be an expression of some genes for some patients [21].

When the vascular is challenged via increased inflammation, monocytes are activated increasing the inflammatory response and promoting alterations in vascular endothelial function. The proximity between EAT and coronary blood vessels makes pro-inflammatory adipokines from epicardial fat to the vascular wall much easier and efficient. In the obesogenic state, EAT cells are enlarged and have an increased production of pro-inflammatory agents, predominately IL6 and TNFα. The ability to communicate with the coronary blood vessels without a barrier allows vasocrine or paracrine cross talk. EAT hypertrophy in patients with obesity or type II diabetes creates a dysfunctional cell and the release of fatty acid with the pro-inflammatory factors. EAT mass and thickness are increased in obesity with a strong correlation with abdominal fat accumulation. EAT enlargement is associated with increased coronary artery calcium scoring [22].

A study of 60 children found cardiac remodeling can begin to occur in children with obesity as young as 8 years old [23]. The Internet 99 study with 6238 adults had findings of obesity being associated with a higher incidence of ischemic heart disease irrespective of metabolic status, leading to the finding that questions the feasibility of denoting a subgroup of individuals with obesity as metabolically healthy [24].

Clinical Implications

The vascular system is highly plastic in nature, and weight loss can partially or completely reverse the deleterious hemodynamic and vascular consequences of obesity. Even though the majority of the book is directed at the treatment of adults, anyone in primary care can see the importance from the cardiovascular data to recognize, diagnose, and begin treatment early for children.

Obesity treatment interventions including bariatric surgery show reductions in EAT. ACEE recommends anti-obesity medications for consideration; orlistat has been shown to reduce adipose tissue volume and decrease LDL, triglycerides, and fasting glucose [3]. EAT showed a 13% decrease with the use of liraglutide in patients with T2DM [25]. And as appropriate assure the patient is on a statin. The amount of EAT reduction cannot be predicted by the overall amount of weight loss, as most impressively demonstrated by the finding that in spite of the much greater reduction in bodyweight that occurred by means of bariatric surgery, EAT decrease was similar to that observed in the group of patients undergoing just dietary intervention. This could suggest that there's a limit on the possible EAT reduction consistent with the need for EAT to retain its physiologic role [25].

There is controversy around weight-loss and cardiovascular disease. In fact, ACEE actually states weight loss therapy is not recommended for the sole purpose of preventing cardiovascular disease or to extend life [3].

Atrial Fibrillation (Afib)

Mechanism

Obesity is correlated with a greater frequency of developing Afib, and the risk factors include structural and electrical remodeling of the atria at both the macro and micro levels. EAT amount contributes to structural and electrical remodeling of the myocardium. The larger amount of EAT presence worsens chronicity, recurrence after ablation and cardioversion, and a symptom burden. EAT also induces fibrosis of the myocardium, through pro-fibrotic mediators and inflammatory cytokines. EAT also increases SNS tone. The hallmark of macroscopic change is atrial dilation. Microscopic changes include cellular hypertrophy, fibrosis, apoptosis, and fatty infiltration. These are thought to contribute to abnormal atrial conduction that favors reentry and endo-epicardial electrical dissociation, both of which can result in afib.

Clinical Implications

A 10% weight loss is associated with the sixfold greater probability of afib free survival as compared to those who didn't lose weight. An absence of weight gain and regain cycle was important [26].

Heart Failure

The obesity connection with heart failure includes the obesity paradox [27]. Higher BMI rates had lower rates of hospitalization and mortality in the study published in the *Archives of Internal Medicine*. Further studies found instead that higher BMI was associated with more severe heart failure bringing the obesity paradox into question. Heo [28] looked at 302 patients and their findings did not support the obesity paradox in relationship between obesity and heart failure symptoms. Higher levels of BMI were associated with more severe heart failure symptoms in both males and females.

Shah's [29] study looked at body mass index in mortality in acutely decompensated heart failure across the world. They looked at 6142 patients with acute decompensated heart failure. Their findings demonstrated the obesity paradox was confined to older persons with decreased cardiac function, less cardiometabolic illness, and new onset heart failure. This suggests that aging heart failure severity and chronicity as well as metabolism may explain the previously reported obesity paradox.

Sharma [30] looked at 22,807 patients. Their finding's total cardiovascular mortality, as well as hospitalization, was highest with underweight patients with chronic heart failure. The risk for cardiovascular mortality at hospitalization was lowest in overweight patients: BMI 25–29.9 kg/m^2. Increasing degree of obesity failed to achieve a statistically significant effect on CV mortality and/or hospitalization.

Clinical Implications

Excess adiposity within limits may reflect a metabolic safety net for catabolic needs and heart failure. Prevention of underweight and obesity in elders with decreased cardiac function would seem to result in fewer comorbidities. The length of time in heart failure may be of importance.

Dyslipidemia

Mechanism

Hypothesis is that high carbohydrate consumption drives hepatic VLDL production. Insulin resistance also elevates triglycerides. HDL becomes dysfunctional due to the inflammation and oxidative stress and the ability to remove cholesterol lowers. HDL clearance occurs faster than production. And there seems to be a downregulation of Apo-A (which removes cholesterol to form HDL). Free fatty acids from adipose tissue increases the amount of VLDL and also leads to more triglycerides. The relationship between BMI and circulating lipids is complex. Insulin and leptin are secreted in direct proportion, and adiponectin in negative proportion, to the size of the adipose mass. All of this creates a circular movement of increasing lipids, then more lipids increase insulin resistance, which increases leptin resistance and adds to increased lipids.

Clinical Implications

Treating obesity with lifestyle therapy including meal planning and minimizing sugar and carbohydrates, avoiding trans fats, and limits of ETOH, as well as increasing physical activity impacts hyperlipidemia. Assuring adequate polyunsaturated fatty acids, like Omega 3 and 6 with decreased triglycerides, is also recommended.

Hypertension

Mechanism

HTN and obesity connection appears to relate to excessive reactive oxygen species production, abnormal RAAS (especially aldosterone), and pro-inflammatory signaling. Specifically, monocytes promote the inflammatory response changing the vascular endothelium. Reduced nitric oxide availability and activity also play a role. The mechanisms causing this vascular dysfunction involves the combined effect of oxidative stress and inflammatory signaling, widely recognized as major players in the pathogenesis of cardiovascular disease. Excessive activity of sympathetic nervous system is a hallmark of obesity, and sympathetic overactivity promotes inflammatory signaling. This occurs through cytokines such as MCP-1, TNFα, and interleukin family of cytokines (IL-1, IL-6, and IL-17).

Insulin resistance and hyperinsulinemia could directly cause hypertension via the increase in catecholamine activity independent of plasma glucose concentrations. Peripheral vascular adipose tissue (PVAT) is a layer of fat tissue that encases the blood vessels and acts as a dynamic endocrine organ. It exerts a differential effect on vascular reactivity. With normal levels of adiposity, the PVAT is primarily anti-contractile. It does this by enhancing nitrous oxide bioavailability within the endothelium. In patients with obesity there is a reduction in NOS expression in vascular tissues. Combine this with the increase in inflammatory markers and increase in oxidative stress and it equals more inflammation. All of this increases the contractile state of the vascular bed. During early stages of obesity nitrous oxide overproduction occurs within the PVAT, perhaps aimed at maintaining vascular function. However, as obesity progresses the previously mentioned things occur, increasing vasoconstriction [31].

Leptin elevation increases SNS activation in the central nervous system as well as receptors in the peripheral endothelium and smooth muscle vasculature, further promotion of inflammation equals the development of arterial wall stiffening. There are increased levels of leptin in circulation likely due to leptin resistance.

Clinical Implications

Weight loss can partially or completely reverse the vascular consequence of obesity even after they occur. Five to fifteen percent weight reduction is generally needed to achieve blood pressure reduction. ACEE [3] recommends any of the AOMS except naltrexone/ bupropion ER and a caution with phentermine/topiramate ER. Blood pressure and heart rate should be closely monitored. Naltrexone/bupropion ER may need to be avoided with uncontrolled hypertension. Bariatric surgery should be considered and Roux-en-Y or the sleeve gastrectomy are the ones recommended.

Polycystic Ovary Syndrome (PCOS) and Female Infertility

Mechanism

Obesity connection with PCOS relates to the hyperinsulinemia, low sex hormone binding globulin (SHBG), and changes to the HPA. Increased insulin levels increase ovarian androgen production. Leptin has a role in ovulation with releasing GnRH from the hypothalamus causing ovulation. But with leptin resistance this is impacted. Adipose tissue causes conversion and increase in estrone which increases endometrial hyperplasia. SHBG decreases causing an increase in bioavailable testosterone. Infertility then is due to anovulation and elevated testosterone.

As previously mentioned, adiponectin is decreased in obesity and is associated with hyperinsulinemia. There is also a decrease in production of hepatic SHBG that's contributing to hyperinsulinism and hyperinsulinemia impacting ovulation through granulosis cell apoptosis [32].

Clinical Implications

Five to ten percent weight loss (although in some patients this will need to be higher) is needed to improve hyperandrogenism, oligomenorrhea, anovulation, insulin resistance, and hyperlipidemia. ACEE [3] recommends treatment with orlistat, metformin, or liraglutide alone or in combination with bariatric surgery.

Male Hypogonadism

We don't want to leave men out of our ORC discussion on fertility☺. Insulin resistance leads to decreased SHBG. Ninety-eight percent of testosterone normally is bound to SHBG and a bit to albumin so only 2% is active. Low binding proteins decrease the bioavailable hormone. Adipose tissue also promotes the conversion of free testosterone to estrogen, adding to testosterone deficiency. Leptin also suppresses gonadal steroidogenesis. The negative feedback from the alteration of testosterone to estrogen ratio may eventually cause a decrease in GnRH (gonadotropin-release hormone), from the hypothalamus, which can alter the LH (luteinizing hormone) amplitude, resulting in lower testosterone levels. Serum testosterone levels decrease with increasing BMI [33].

Clinical Implications

Weight loss of 5–10% will start to demonstrate improvement in serum testosterone. When clinically evaluating patients with obesity, it is important to identify specific signs of hypogonadism, including low libido, decreased morning erection, loss of body hair, gynecomastia, and small testes. Most useful screening tests are both serum total testosterone, where possible measured by mass spectrometry, and calculated free testosterone from total testosterone.

Testosterone replacement should only be considered when true biochemical and clinical evidence of hypogonadism. Advantages are weight loss, decreased waist circumference, improved muscle strength, free fat mass, bone density, and metabolic parameters. The risks include sleep apnea, cardiovascular disease, and deep vein thrombosis.

Practice Pearls

- Treating obesity treats many other diseases seen and treated in primary care (Table 5.2).
- As little as 5% weight loss in obesity treatment can impact other chronic diseases or delay them.
- The complications alone can explain obesity as a disease.

TABLE 5.2 Complication of obesity, mechanism, and clinical implication

Disease	Mechanism based on obesity	Clinical implication for treatment
Cancer	Increased hormones Increased leptin Chronic inflammation	Weight loss = 20% reduction in all-cause mortality Due to bias and stigma patients avoid healthcare = later stage recognition
NALFD	Ectopic fat deposition in the liver Chronic inflammation	7% weight loss can improve steatosis May require 40% for histologic improvement
ORG	Ectopic fat deposition in the kidney Inflammation and oxidative stress activates RAAS	Weight loss can prevent chronic kidney disease or further damage if scarring has occurred
CKD	Ectopic fat deposition Increased filtration and intraglomerular pressure	Weight loss can reduce hyperfiltration Use of RAAS blockage medications to support the kidney Consider SGLT-2 if treating DM
Prediabetes/ diabetes/ metabolic syndrome	Increased free fatty acids Ectopic fat deposition in muscle, kidneys, and pancreas	Treating obesity can prevent risk of T2DM, 10% weight loss reduces T2DM risk by 80%

(continued)

Table 5.2 (continued)

Disease	Mechanism based on obesity	Clinical implication for treatment
Atrial fibrillation	Structural and electrical remodeling with ectopic fat deposit Increased EAT worsens chronicity and recurrence	10% weight loss is predictive of preventing recurrence of afib Weight loss and weight regain cycles are important in preventing recurrence of afib
Dyslipidemia	Increased VLDL production Insulin resistance Inflammation and oxidative stress	Treatment of obesity impacts all dyslipidemia factors
Hypertension	Excessive reactive oxygen species Abnormal RAAS Pro-inflammation Increased SNS activity	5–15% weight loss can partially or completely reverse vascular consequences of obesity
PCOS	Increased ovarian androgen production Endometrial hyperplasia Low sex hormone binding globulin Changes to HPA	5–10% weight loss can improve anovulation, hyperandrogenism, oligomenorrhea, insulin resistance, and dyslipidemia
Hypogonadism	Decreased SHBG Decreased bioavailability of testosterone Decreased serum testosterone	5–10% weight loss improves serum testosterone

Conclusion

It seemed important to use these examples of how obesity impacts diseases being treated every day in primary care. So a question that I heard asked at a conference: "How can I add one more thing to what I am doing" and the answer I heard from an NP expert in obesity, Chris Kessler, October 2019, "How can you NOT make time to treat obesity when it underlies so much of what takes the time in primary care? And by treating obesity you are treating so many other diseases and disorders or potentially even preventing them thereby saving time in the long run."

References

1. Yeun M, Earle R, Kadambi N, Brancale J, Lui D, Kahan S, Kaplan L. A systematic review and evaluation of current evidence reveals 236 obesity-associated disorders (ObAD). Poster presented at: Obesity Week Conference of the Obesity Society. New Orleans; 2016.
2. Heymsfield SB, Wadden TA. Mechanisms, pathophysiology and management of obesity. N Engl J Med. 2017;376(3):254–66.
3. Garvey WT, Mechanick JI, Brett EM, Garber AJ, Hurley DL, Jastreboff AM, Reviewers of the AACE/ACE Obesity Clinical Practice Guidelines, et al. American Association of Clinical Endocrinologists and American College of Endocrinology comprehensive clinical practice guidelines for medical care of patients with obesity. Endocr Pract. 2016;22(S3):1–203.
4. American Association of Clinical Endocrinologists. Treatment algorithm for the medical care of patients with obesity. 2016. https://www.aace.com/disease-state-resources/nutrition-and-obesity/treatment-algorithms/treatment-algorithm-medical-care. Accessed 11 Apr 2020.
5. Zheng Y, Manson J, Yuan C, Liang M, Grodstein F, Stampfer M, et al. Associations of eight gain from early to middle adult-hood with major health outcomes later in life. JAMA. 2017;318(3):255–69.

6. American Association for Cancer Research. 2018. https://www.cancerprogressreport.org/Pages/default.aspx. Accessed 11 Apr 2020.
7. Parekh N, Lin Y, Vadiveloo M, Hayes R, Lu-Yao G. Metabolic dysregulation of the insulin–glucose axis and risk of obesity-related cancers in the framingham heart study-offspring cohort (1971–2008). Cancer Epidemiol Biomarkers Prev. 2013;22(10):1825–36.
8. Arnold M, Jiang L, Stefanick M, Johnson K, Lane D, LeBlanc E, et al. Duration of adulthood overweight, obesity, and cancer risk in the women's health initiative: a longitudinal study from the United States. PLoS Med. 2016;13(8):e1002081. https://doi.org/10.1371/journal.pmed.100208.
9. Targher G, Byrne C. Nonalcoholic fatty liver disease: a novel cardiometabolic risk factor for type 2 diabetes and its complications. J Clin Endocrinol Metab. 2013;98(2):483–95.
10. Bzowej N. Nonalcoholic steatohepatitis: the frontier for liver transplantation. Curr Opin Organ Transplant. 2018;23(2):169–74.
11. Ryan M, Itsiopoulos C, Thodis T, Ward G, Tros N, Hofferberth S, O'Dea K, Desmond P, Johnson N, Wilson A. The Mediterranean diet improves hepatic steatosis and insulin sensitivity in individuals with non-alcoholic fatty liver disease. J Hepatol. 2013;59(1):138–43.
12. Vizuete J, Camero A, Malakouti M, Garapati K, Gutierrez J. Perspectives on nonalcoholic fatty liver disease: an overview of present and future therapies. J Clin Transl Hepatol. 2017;5(1):67–75.
13. Camara N, Iseki K, Kramer H, Liu Z, Sharma K. Kidney disease and obesity: epidemiology, mechanisms and treatment. Nat Rev Nephrol. 2017;13:181–90.
14. D'Agati V, Chagnac A, de Vries A, Levi M, Porrini E, Herman-Edelstein M, Praga M. Obesity-related glomerulopathy: clinical and pathologic characteristics and pathogenesis. Nat Rev Nephrol. 2016;12(8):453–71. https://doi.org/10.1038/nrneph.2016.75.
15. Kovesdy C, Furth S, Zoccali C. Obesity and kidney disease: hidden consequences of epidemic. Clin Kidney J. 2017;10(1):1–8.
16. World Health Organization. About diabetes. n.d. https://www.who.int/diabetes/action_online/basics/en/index2.html. Accessed 11 Apr 2020.
17. Shuchleib-Cung A, Akusoba I, Higa K. Diabesity: the worldwide twin epidemics of obesity and diabetes. Bariatric Times. 2018;15(9):14–20.

18. Flegal KM, Kruszon-Moran D, Carroll MD, Fryar CD, Ogden CL. Trends in obesity among adults in the United States, 2005 to 2014. JAMA. 2016;315(21):2284–91.
19. Lee YS, Kim JW, Osborne O, Sasik R, Schenk S, Chen A, Watkins SM, Quehenberger O, Johnson RS, Olefsky JM. Increased adipocyte O2 consumption triggers HIF-1α, causing inflammation and insulin resistance in obesity. Cell. 2014;157(6):1339–52. https://doi.org/10.1016/j.cell.2014.05.012.
20. Goossens GH, Blaak EE. Adipose tissue dysfunction and impaired metabolic health in human obesity: a matter of oxygen? Front Endocrinol. 2015;6(55):1–5.
21. Ormazabal V, Nair S, Elfeky O, Aguayo C, Salomon C, Zuñiga F. Association between insulin resistance and the development of cardiovascular disease. Cardiovasc Diabetol. 2018;17(122):1–14. https://doi.org/10.1186/s12933-018-0762-4.
22. Salazar J, Luzardo E, Mejias J, Rojas J, Ferreira A, Rivas-Rios J, Bermudez V. Epicardial fat: physiological, pathological, and therapeutic implications. Cardiol Res Pract. 2016;2016:1291537. https://doi.org/10.1155/2016/1291537.
23. Jing L, Binkley C, Suever J, Umasankar N, Haggerty C, Nevius C, et al. Cardiac remodeling and dysfunction in childhood obesity: a cardiovascular magnetic resonance study. J Cardiovasc Magn Reson. 2016;18:28):1–12.
24. Jansen L, Netterstrom M, Johansen N, Ronn P, Vistisen D, Husemoen N, et al. Metabolically healthy obesity and ischemic heart disease: a 10-year follow-up of the Inter99 study. J Clin Endocrinol Metab. 2017;102(6):1934–42.
25. Gonzalez N, Moreno-Villegas Z, Gonzalez-Bris A, Egido J, Lorenzo O. Regulation of visceral and epicardial adipose tissue for preventing cardiovascular injuries associated to obesity and diabetes. Cardiovasc Diabetol. 2017;16:44. https://doi.org/10.1186/s12933-017-0528-4.
26. Mahajan R, Pathak R, Thiyagarajah A, Lau D, Marchlinski F, Dixit S, et al. Risk factor management and atrial fibrillation clinics: saving the best for last? Heart Lung Circ. 2017;26(9):990–7. https://doi.org/10.1016/j.hlc.2017.05.123.
27. Curtis J, Selter J, Wang Y, Rathore S, Jovin I, Jadbabaie F, et al. The obesity paradox: body mass index and outcomes in patients with heart failure. Arch Intern Med. 2005;165(1):55–61. https://doi.org/10.1001/archinte.165.1.55.

28. Heo S, Moser DK, Pressler SJ, Dunbar SB, Lee KS, Kim J, Lennie TA. Association between obesity and heart failure symptoms in male and female patients. Clin Obes. 2017;7:77–85. https://doi.org/10.1111/cob.12179.
29. Shah R, Gayat E, Januzzi JL, Sato N, Cohen-Solal A, di Somma S, et al. Body mass index and mortality in acutely decompensated heart failure across the world: a global obesity paradox. J Am Coll Cardiol. 2014;63(8):778–85. https://doi.org/10.1016/j.jacc.2013.09.072.
30. Sharma A, Lavie CJ, Borer JS, Vallakati A, Goel S, Lopez-Jimenez F, et al. Meta-analysis of the relation of body mass index to all-cause and cardiovascular mortality and hospitalization in patients with chronic heart failure. Am J Cardiol. 2015;115(10):1428–38. https://doi.org/10.1016/j.amjcard.2015.o2.024. Epub 18 Feb 2015.
31. Fernández-Alfonso MS, Gil-Ortega M, García-Prieto CF, Arangue I, Ruiz-Gayo M, Somoza B. Mechanisms of perivascular adipose tissue dysfunction in obesity. Int J Endocrinol. 2013;2013:402053. https://doi.org/10.1155/2013/402053.
32. Rojas J, Chávez M, Olivar L, Rojas M, Morillo J, Mejías J, et al. Polycystic ovary syndrome, insulin resistance, and obesity: navigating the pathophysiologic labyrinth. Int J Reprod Med. 2014;2014:719050. https://doi.org/10.1155/2014/719050.
33. Poddar M, Chetty Y, Chetty VT. How does obesity affect the endocrine system? A narrative review. Clin Obes. 2017;7:136–44.

Part II
Building a Treatment Plan

Evaluating obesity in the chronic disease model will provide primary care with a structure that is familiar to clinical practice. This section will then look at the evidence-based practice recommendations for the foundational components of the treatment plan of eating plans, physical activity and behavior interventions. Following the foundation treatment, the supportive treatment of medication and/or procedures and devices will be discussed.

Introduction to Part Two

As the process of building a treatment plan begins let's take one moment to remember that many people say the problem with the increasing incidence of obesity is just that we are eating more. Ford [1] shows through the trends in energy intake he clearly demonstrates that there has not been a dramatic increase in calories overtime. This helps guide us to recognize the multifactorial approach in treating obesity. The Obesity Medicine Association lists 4 pillars for obesity treatment: Eating, Activity, Behavior, Medication. I would suggest we combine the evidenced based guidelines and use three foundational components; Eating plans, Physical Activity, and Behavior Interventions with two supportive components; medications and procedures/surgeries (Table P2.1). Medications, procedures and surgeries still require the initial

TABLE P2.1 Comparison of pillars and components conceptually

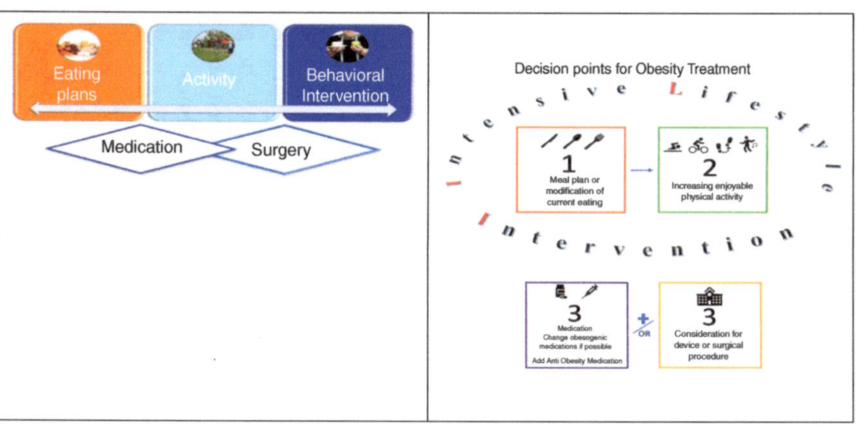

basis of treatment to be successful but can support the foundation components to provide greater success.

Reference

1. Ford E, Dietz W. Trends in energy intake among adults in the United States: findings from NHANES. Am J Clin Nutr. 2013;97(4):848–53.

Chapter 6
Chronic Disease Model for Obesity

EFFICIENCY IS DOING THE THING RIGHT,
EFFECTIVENESS IS DOING THE RIGHT THING.

PETER DRUCKER

Key Reason
Integrating obesity treatment into a practice can feel overwhelming; however, the case has been made that it must be done. This chapter is designed to identify barriers and solutions for integration.

Introduction

This chapter examines the role of the chronic care model which is a multifactorial care delivery system. The utilization of this model with the chronic disease of obesity in primary care is explored. There are many barriers to adding something else into an already busy primary care practice. Overcoming these barriers is essential to treating obesity in primary care.

Every practice understands that treating chronic diseases through a collaborative model of care has been well

A. Golden, *Treating Obesity in Primary Care*,
https://doi.org/10.1007/978-3-030-48683-9_6

Table 6.1 Barriers to implementing obesity into primary care

Barriers to implementing obesity into primary care
Number of patients to treat
Lack of education about what the disease is (and isn't) in your practice for individuals and the overall practice or healthcare system
Being unaware of the available national guidelines to use to guide treatment
Lack of access to multidisciplinary teams
Systematic process for making the diagnosis
Opening the conversation

documented. However, before we discuss what the chronic care model is and how to apply it to obesity in various practice/system settings, we need to acknowledge a few of the barriers to managing obesity as a chronic disease in this systematic model (Table 6.1). The first may simply be the overwhelming numbers. With almost 40% of the adult population already having the disease of obesity, this can seem overwhelming to add to your busy practice. Of course, we can't ignore it—so much of what we are treating in primary care is directly caused or associated with this disease. So, let's just be honest that we may not *want* to add one more thing to our day and set this aside as we realize we just have to do it. After all, if you are reading this book, you are likely interested in how you can best help your patients.

Many research articles have demonstrated that very few healthcare providers graduating today (let alone in the past) have any education about obesity (or even treating people with "excess weight") beyond the eat less move more paradigm. With the complexity of this disease we know that the eat less move more advise is ineffective. And oh, by the way every patient has already tried, often more than seven times before talking with you [1].

For most of us in primary care don't have easy access to multidisciplinary professionals as demonstrated in the chronic care model. Many primary care practices are small without the additional providers such as dieticians, behaviorists, and exercise physiologist, this can feel like a large barrier.

Another barrier is actually making the diagnosis to acknowledge the disease exists. It is hard to treat something even in the best chronic disease model if you haven't diagnosed it. Research clearly shows that as clinicians we aren't doing this [1]. Once diagnosed many providers are uncomfortable opening the conversation; without a discussion no chronic care model will do much of anything for your patients. Again, since you are reading the book you get all this, but you can help your colleagues do a better job and therefore help more patients. So, let's make the diagnosis and start the conversation with our patients and look at a model that you may have in place for other diseases and can adapt to obesity.

The definition of a chronic disease is a long-lasting condition that can be controlled but not cured. Chronic disease models have three phases of intervention: primary, secondary, and tertiary (Table 6.2) [2].

Chronic Care Model

The chronic care model (CCM) is a multifactorial care delivery system that is an evidence-based framework for improving the delivery of care [3]. Essential components of the healthcare system should be modified to support high-quality, patient-centered chronic disease management. Elements of the CCM include health systems, decision support, clinical information system, patient self-management community resources, and a system design to deliver clinical care [4]. The CCM process calls for a structural change in the way people with chronic illnesses are cared for with multidisciplinary teams and the patient as the center of the team [5].

Many chronic diseases are now managed and treated in primary care with diabetes, hyperlipidemia, and hypertension to name just a few. The strategies being used for this are var-

TABLE 6.2 Chronic care model prevention

Phase	Intervention	Relate to obesity	Methods
Primary	Education of the general public looking at the environment and promote healthy living	Prevent both overweight and obesity from occurring	Community education Policy Advocacy
Secondary	Prevent further progression of a disease or complications in an individual	Prevent future progression of obesity for an individual and prevent the development of obesity-related complications	Screening using a BMI at every visit—if positive screening moving to diagnosis Waist circumference with diagnosis—treating obesity with lifestyle and behavioral interventions and as appropriate anti-obesity medications and/or a referral to bariatric surgery program
Tertiary	Increasing treatment for disease and complications	Aggressive treatment of obesity to eliminate or reduce the complications related to obesity and to continue to prevent the progression of the disease of obesity	Assuring treatment is in place for obesity and complications May need consultation with obesity specialist or bariatrician

ied depending on the model being used, but all have similarities, and all have the goal of improving clinical outcomes for patients. There are general concepts in all chronic care models that include the support of the organization where the clinician works, a designed program of care, self-management for the patient that is supported, and the use of community resources (Table 6.3). It is easy to see how obesity treatment fits in this process.

Table 6.3 Chronic care model for practices without full multidisciplinary teams

Concept	Primary care	Specific issues
Organizational support	Scanning and changing potential bias in the practice	Bias tests Appropriate equipment Education about the disease for all staff
Program of care	Consistent approach to treatment of the disease by all staff	Maximizing utilization of all staff members for treatment of obesity Utilizing evidence-based guidelines Decision support processes—finding specialists that understand the disease for referrals, reminder systems for patient follow-ups Evaluating need for practice improvement by evaluating outcomes Using ready make programs, for example, Diabetes Prevention Program as an outline for an obesity program. Canadian Obesity Network program – 5As is designed for primary care and treatment of obesity

(continued)

TABLE 6.3 (continued)

Concept	Primary care	Specific issues
Self-management	Assuring patient feels supported by all staff members	Patient-centered—meaning patient is central to goal decisions—setting priorities, identifying barriers, and creating plans to remove barriers Use motivational interviewing in practice to assist with problem-solving, decision-making Utilizing available resources Positive patient and provider relationship
Community resources	Determining community resources Assuring they understand the disease of obesity	Dieticians with Interdisciplinary Specialist Certification in Obesity and Weight Management credential Talk to the exercise professionals in your community and find physical therapists or fitness coaches that understand the disease of obesity Other examples of community resources: Peer support organizations (e.g., silver sneakers at the YMCA or YWCA: farmers markets that make fresh vegetables available (some even accept food stamps) Caution: referral to a community resource that will create more shame or is biased will create a barrier to treatment

Practice Pearls

- Having a chronic care model does not require a large health system, you can create one using your own practice and community services.
- In a large health system, it may be harder to assure that bias and stigma are not occurring in other areas of the practice the patient is interacting.
- No matter the system, the patient must be at the center and part of all decision-making.

References

1. Kaplan LM, Golden A, Jinnett K, Kolotkin RL, Kyle TK, Look M, et al. Perceptions of barriers to effective obesity care: results from the national ACTION study. Obesity. 2016;26:61. https://doi.org/10.1002/oby.22054.
2. Siminerio L, Zgibor J, Solano F. Implementing the chronic care model for improvements in diabetes practice and outcomes in primary care: the University of Pittsburgh Medical Center experience. Clin Diabetes. 2004;22:54–8.
3. Coleman K, Austin B, Brach C, Wagner E. Evidence on the chronic care model in the new millennium. Health Aff. 2009;28(1):75–85.
4. Grover A, Joshi A. An overview of chronic disease models: a systematic literature review. Global J Health Sci. 2014;7(2):210–27.
5. Fiandt K. The chronic care model: description and application for practice. Top Adv Pract Nurs. 2006;6(4):6.

Chapter 7
Evidence-Based Guidelines for the Treatment of Obesity

EVEN IF YOU'RE ON THE RIGHT TRACK YOU'LL GET RUN OVER IF YOU JUST SIT STILL.

WILL ROGERS

Key Reason
All of the chronic diseases we currently treat have national or international guideline to help guide our treatment decisions. Obesity does as well. Due to all the non-evidence based treatment being offered in the "over-the-counter" options and even by our healthcare peers it is critical that we are all familiar with the guidance being provided by the national guidelines.

Introduction

This chapter examines the evidence-based guidelines available for the disease of obesity. Brief overview of each guideline with the emphasis of that guideline is reviewed. A summary of the components of treatment as addressed by the guidelines is also included.

A. Golden, *Treating Obesity in Primary Care*,
https://doi.org/10.1007/978-3-030-48683-9_7

There are numerous guidelines available for clinicians. A discussion of using them in primary care is critical to the success of assisting patients in treating obesity. Every guideline starts with the foundational treatment. The foundational components include helping a patient find an eating plan they can maintain, ways to increase physical activity, and the use of behavioral interventions to partner with patients to be successful with the first two components in the treatment of obesity. From that point on the guidelines have some nuances to consider in practice which we will review.

Another aspect that all of the guidelines have in common is they are concentrating on a comprehensive approach to the treatment of obesity recognizing the importance of the obesity-related complications and how treating obesity can improve those. All of the guidelines emphasize the chronic nature of obesity and its relapsing nature thus stressing long-term treatment is needed, just like for diabetes. The guidelines also recommend referrals to an obesity specialist if the patient is struggling and/or unable to meet their goals.

As guidelines have advanced the recommendations go beyond treatment of lifestyle and introduce the use of pharmacology and/or surgery. These also put an emphasis on treating obesity as a part of a comprehensive and multidisciplinary treatment plan focusing on the goal of 5–10% weight loss. This goal is due to the effect on the complications and comorbidities associated with obesity. Patients, however, often have a different "number" than the guideline recommendations.

Other commonalities in the guidelines are the use of BMI as a *screening* measure but not the only measure to determine diagnosis and therefore treatment. The three guidelines agree that patients with excess adiposity, regardless of BMI, who have health risks or complications of obesity should be treated for obesity.

AHA/ACC/TOS [1] guideline recommends that all patients with a BMI over 30 (with a cut off of 25 for Asians) should be treated with medical treatment of obesity with a minimum of intensive weight loss interventions. The rationale this states is that even without a complication those patients will likely progress overtime to have complications and/or comorbid conditions.

Although the guidelines recommend comprehensive lifestyle intervention as the cornerstone of the three components in clinical practice, most patients have already been doing this through self-help approach or have been in community-based programs. Now not all of those have been appropriate (i.e., cabbage soup diet) but patients have been trying with non-sustained attempts at self-treating. Therefore, in clinical practice it is likely that we are initiating pharmacology early in the treatment plan.

Table of obesity guidelines lists the available guidelines in the United States (Table 7.1). This chapter will refer primarily to three guidelines (Table 7.2) and one algorithm to assist in

Table 7.1 Obesity guideline brief overview and reference site

Guideline/ organization	Brief overview	Guideline reference
AHA/ACC/ TOS	Comprehensive guideline covering the evidence as of 2012 with emphasis on eating, activity, behavior therapy, pharmacology, and medications	https://www.ahajournals.org/doi/full/10.1161/01.cir.0000437739.71477.ee
AACE, TOS, and ASMBS	The guideline reviews the importance of the three pillars (eating, activity, and behavior) as well as the recommendations for pre- and post-op care for patients getting surgery	https://www.ncbi.nlm.nih.gov/pmc/articles/PMC4142593/

(continued)

Table 7.1 (continued)

Guideline/ organization	Brief overview	Guideline reference
VA/DoD	Includes the basics of treatment, with recommendations for pharmacology and surgery. This guideline provides additional information on use of generics and items that should not be used	https://www.healthquality.va.gov/guidelines/cd/obesity/
Endocrine Society	Overview of available pharmacology and an important history of decreasing the number of obesogenic medications	https://academic.oup.com/jcem/article/100/2/342/28131
AACE/ACE	This guideline is complication based for treatment recommendations	http://obesity.aace.com/medical_society_guidelines_for_treatment_of_obesity
OMA	Comprehensive review of current evidence for eating plans, physical activity recommendations, and behavioral therapy. Incudes pharmacology recommendations and appropriate referral to surgical programs	https://obesitymedicine.org/obesity-algorithm/ (has a cost involved if not a member); https://obesitymedicine.org/obesity-algorithm/download-now/ (no charge but must complete registration)

Table 7.2 Guideline overview related to components of treatment

Eating	Guide to understand various eating plans, no one plan will work for everyone with obesity	When your patient is making a decision it has to be the eating plan with the patient feels they have the best chance of staying with. This is a perfect example of shared decision-making
Physical activity	Goal during active treatment 150 minutes/week, increasing to 200–300 minutes/week in maintenance	The first step is getting your patient to move
Medication	Explain use and safety of medications, use with specific obesity related complications	Begin to evaluate the appropriate use of medication during the intake history and physical

guiding treatment in clinic. The three guidelines are the 2013 AHA/ACC/TOS [1] Guidelines for Managing Overweight and Obesity in Adults, 2015 Endocrine Society [2] Pharmacologic Management of Obesity: An Endocrine Society Clinical Practice Guideline, and the 2016 AACE/ACE [3] Obesity Clinical Practice Guideline. Obesity Medicine Association [4] updates the Obesity Algorithm every year or two. AHA/ACC/TOS [1] and Endocrine Society [2] use systematic evidence review with graded recommendations, while OMA and AACE/ACE do literature reviews and then expert consensus.

Guidelines and Eating

One of the issues around treating obesity is which eating plan should be used for which patient or is there just one eating plan that works for everyone. Many studies have looked at all the different macronutrient compositions. Of course, the one that's been around for a very long time is the low-fat diet; currently low carbohydrate seems to be the most common one that can be found on the Internet as the answer to all the treatment of obesity and weight-loss. In the AHA/ACC/TOS [1] guidelines there's a systematic review of 17 different dietary patterns. This review clearly demonstrates there is no one eating plan for every patient. The best predictor of success in obesity treatment with an eating plan is long-term adherence.

Guidelines and Physical Activity

Looking at the guidelines on physical activity, it is an essential part of the comprehensive lifestyle intervention. Be sure to assess if it is safe for a patient to increase activity and then move forward. The guidelines suggest that there be brisk aerobic physical activity that equals 150 minutes or more each week, or the equivalency of 10,000 steps a day. This will need to increase to 200–300 minutes or more each week for maintenance. There is also the issue of resistance training. There was no evidence that resistance training directly improves outcomes in the active phase of treatment. However, resistance training does have benefits: patients can increase fat-free mass and this is associated with reductions in health risks. So, the importance of aerobic and anaerobic exercise is it can improve a person's overall health and decrease the risk of other diseases.

Guidelines and Medications

The Endocrine Society [2] guideline is really the first authority. This guideline recommends during the history to be looking for obesogenic medications that may need to be changed for patients. This guideline also provides recommendations for medications that are either weight neutral, less obesogenic, or could actually support the treatment of obesity with weight loss. What this guideline doesn't do is provide any indication of which anti-obesity medications to start first. This guideline strongly recommends that medication is only effective when combined with intensive lifestyle interventions. This matches the labels of each of the medications. AACE guideline and their obesity resource center does provide guidance on specific anti-obesity medications but is based on the obesity-related complication.

Specific to AHA/ACC/TOS [1]

- Does not have the complete information for medication management (due to publication date)
- Excellent information on the evidence basis for the foundational components with eating plans, physical activity and behavior interventions
- Recommendation of when to refer for bariatric surgery due to substantial amount of total body weight reduction and the improvement or reversal of obesity related complications and comorbidities

Specific to AACE/ACE [5]

- Approaches obesity treatment based on severity of disease
- Primary treatment is prevention and should be offered to every patient—teaching every patient healthy eating and managing physical activity
- Individualization of treatment is stressed as is chronicity
- Stage 0 begins the secondary treatment—foundational components and consideration of pharmacotherapy
- Stage one and two require tertiary treatment in order to achieve enough weight loss to either reverse the complications or to prevent further deterioration – foundational components and pharmacotherapy (not a consideration), consider bariatric surgery

The guideline also discusses the importance of public policy and health education around environmental changes to support healthy behaviors. It also has treatment based on the clinical goals with the primary endpoint being improvement in obesity-related complications, versus just a decrease in body weight [1]. This guideline provides evidence and background for choosing eating plans, type of physical activity, and behavioral intervention approaches. AACE/ACE [5] recommends a multidisciplinary approach and lists many providers that can be part of a team approach. Additionally, ongoing follow-up, reevaluation, and long-term treatment are needed since obesity is a chronic relapsing disease.

AACE/ACE [5] has a path for when to initiate anti-obesity medications. The first path is for patients with the diagnosis of overweight or obesity who do not yet have any clinically significant obesity-related complications. For these patients, initiating anti-obesity medications would occur if there has been failure on lifestyle therapy. [Authors PEARL: Keep in mind the majority of patients in our practices have already attempted lifestyle therapy, in fact an average of 5–7 times] [1]. The second path for initiation of pharmacology is for patients who have mild-to-moderate complications, weight regain, or lifestyle interventions alone and didn't achieve treatment outcomes. In the last path with the presence of severe obesity-related complications, medication with lifestyle therapy should be initiated early.

Specific to Endocrine Society [2]

- Guideline specifically around medication management
- Starts with a review for obesogenic medications and suggestions for other less obesogenic medications
- Stresses pharmacology as an adjunct to foundational components of treatment

Specific to Obesity Medicine Association [4]

- The OMA aligns with the AACE/ACE and ES guidelines in treatment, but not in diagnosis.
- Uses BMI, WC, and Fat% as diagnosis and staging is based on BMI Stage 1–3.
- Available in an e-book format to make this easier to utilize for clinicians.
- Unique section is reducing bias and shame for patients with obesity.

Summary

As with many other chronic diseases the specialty organizations provide primary care clinicians with a roadmap for the treatment of obesity. There are many similarities between the guidelines and algorithm that provide the basis of the individualized care patients with obesity require.

Practice Pearls
- Recognize national guidelines exist.
- Individualize the treatment based on patient's medical history and past obesity history.
- Recognizing that there is greater urgency with the need for more aggressive therapy if the patient has complications and/or comorbidities with obesity.
- Patients do not need to "fail" with the foundational components or have a lack of success in order to move to treatment with pharmacology and/or surgery.

References

1. Jensen MD, Ryan DH, Apovian CM, Ard JD, Comuzzle AG, Donato KA. AHA/ACC/TOS guideline for the management of overweight and obesity in adults: a report of the American College of Cardiology/American Heart Association task force on practice guidelines and The Obesity Society. Circulation. 2013;129:S102–38. https://doi.org/10.1161/01.cir.0000437739.71477.ee.
2. Apovian CM, Aronne LJ, Bessesen DH, McDonnell ME, Murad MH, Pagotto U, et al. Pharmacological management of obesity: an endocrine society clinical practice guideline. J Clin Endocrinol Metab. 2015;100(2):342–62.
3. Mechanick JI, Youdim A, Jones DB, Garvey WT, Hurley DL, McMahon M, et al. Clinical practice guidelines for the perioperative nutritional, metabolic, and nonsurgical support of the bariatric surgery patient – 2013 update: cosponsored by American Association of Clinical Endocrinologists, The Obesity Society, and American Society for Metabolic & Bariatric Society. Obesity. 2013;21(1):S1–27.

4. Bays HE, McCarthy W, Christensen S, Tondt J, Karjoo S, Davisson L, et al. Obesity algorithm eBook, presented by the Obesity Medicine Association. www.obesityalgorithm.org. 2020. https://obesitymedicine.org/obesity-algorithm/. Accessed 11 Apr 2020.
5. American Association of Clinical Endocrinologists. Treatment algorithm for the medical care of patients with obesity. 2016. https://www.aace.com/disease-state-resources/nutrition-and-obesity/treatment-algorithms/treatment-algorithm-medical-care. Accessed 11 Apr 2020.

Chapter 8
Foundational Component of Treating Obesity: Eating Plans

COURAGE DOESN'T ALWAYS ROAR. SOMETIMES COURAGE IS THE QUIET VOICE AT THE END OF THE DAY SAYING 'I WILL TRY AGAIN TOMORROW.'

MARY ANNE RADMACHER

Key Reason
The first foundational component of treating obesity is changing the way people interact with food. Helping patients understand the impact of food, not just in quantity, on their health is a key to successful treatment.

Introduction

This chapter examines the use of food as a treatment modality. A review of the basic concept of calories, types of calories, and brain regulation of hunger and satiety is completed. Completing an assessment of a patient's eating habits is examined. Overview of various eating plans that can be used to treat obesity is examined with a review of which plan may benefit a specific patient.

A. Golden, *Treating Obesity in Primary Care*,
https://doi.org/10.1007/978-3-030-48683-9_8

Food is a treatment modality. Most obesity experts consider it the first component or pillar of treatment. The component is probably one of the hardest for primary care providers. It takes time to determine patients' current eating patterns and then explain different eating plans to help them select one they can follow or select goals for change in current eating. After all, we all agree now that this is a severe, chronic, relapsing disease so a quick fix won't be the answer. One thing to keep in mind is that the vast majority of our patients have "dieted" so many times in their lives and they don't want to diet again. That is good, and you can use that to your advantage as you talk about long-term treatment for long-term success.

There are a lot of options available for working with food as a prescription, but first we must understand the physiology of hunger and satiety. There are internal and external cues for eating. Internal cues related to homeostasis, neural, nutrient, and hormonal signals communicate with the gut, pancreas, liver, adipose tissue brainstem, and hypothalamus. The arcuate nucleus of the hypothalamus integrates these signals and regulates hunger and satiety in response to the signals via higher cortical centers.

External cues are hedonic and regulated by the corticolimbic system. This system is our "liking and wanting" or rewarding of food. Examples of these are cues that influence intake can be advertising, a personal schedule, and cultural events. This is an example of the hedonic system demonstrated when people report being full but continue to eat dessert.

Selecting an eating plan starts with taking an eating history and determining where the patients is starting from on current eating. My fantasy patient is one that comes into the practice with a daily caloric intake of 3500 calories, eating at fast food places 15 times a week, and drinking 96 ounces of sugar sodas a day. Easy to see where to start for this patient, but this is a fantasy patient for a reason, who probably doesn't exist. More realistic is a patient that is eating a lot less calories, and it may not be so easy for the patient to change, so take it slow in those changes—incremental changes over the long term.

Energy Balance Versus Quality Aka Quantity Versus Quality

The Academy of Nutrition and Dietetics [1] have stated that you need a negative energy balance. OMA, AACE, ACE as organizations and their guidelines have a specific amount of 500 kcal deficit per day. If a patient strictly follows this, they will lose 52 pounds over the next year—RIGHT? We all know that the answer sadly is NO.

Before you take this on for your patients keep in mind that many patients have been "dieting" with weight loss and weight gain for years. I frequently see patients with caloric intake of 1300 kcal/day. It isn't realistic to have them consider 800 kcal for long term unless they are going to use a very low-calorie eating plan under supervision, and even then, this is not a long-term solution.

But before we go further into this, let's see if 3500 kcal deficit leads to 1 pound of weight loss (ideally adipose tissue). The origin of the 3500 kcal per pound rule is misapplied to predict weight change over time after a given intervention. In 1958 a physician, Max Wishnofsky, put forward the concept that 1 pound of fat stored ~3500 kcal. He based this on a pound of fat removed from a patient weighs 454 g and is 87% fat. Thus this pound of fat when doing the math of caloric value (395 × 9.5 = 3750 calories) with the body then having 9 g of fat for energy reserve, thus the 3500 calories = 1 pound of fat [2]. In 2012, American Society for Nutrition and the International Life Sciences Institute panel of experts recommended that the 3500 kcal per pound rule should no longer be used [3]. Newly developed dynamic energy balance models for weight loss require complex calculations that can be simplified using a web-based program (see references).

The scale of energy models helps to demonstrate that the historical thought that obesity is simply calories in and calories out is inaccurate. So here is another example, a patient starts walking to expend 100 kcal/day. Given the 3500 kcal rule, using calories in and calories out, if there is no increase in calories taken in, the patient should see a loss of 50 pounds over 5 years. However, the BWI simulator demonstrates the more likely scenario of 10-pound weight loss over 5 years. So now we have all the evidence we need that this is much more complex than "just" decreasing calories or increasing calories "burned" over the long run. There is a significant metabolic adaptation in energy expenditure as people lose weight.

Let's look at one more concept that we have to consider in primary care. What about the food labels – this might be a surprise but the FDA allows a 20% error on labels [4]. So let's add that up—a patient is eating a food with a label that says 120 calories in a serving, this could mean that the serving is in 100 calories or 132 calories. Now consider that a daily calorie consumption of 2000 calories could be 1600–2400 calories. Think about this over the next year and there could be a great difference in the patient's consumption.

Eating Plans

Dansinger [5] and colleagues did the A to Z study. Their study showed no observable differences among the four diets they looked at Atkins, Ornish, Weight Watchers, and Zone diets. In fact, they found that some patients gained, and some patients lost on each of the eating plan.

Assessment

There are several ways to do an assessment of eating habits. A 24-hour diet recall, 3-day diary, or tracking in an app (Table 8.1). My preference is for a week of an app like My Fitness Pal or Noom.

So, what does this mean for our care of patients with obesity? The first step is to look for modifiable changes with your patient. Examples are limited access to fruits and veg-

TABLE 8.1 Dietary history methods

Method	Pros	Cons
24-hour diet recall	Small burden to patient, literacy is not required	Requires recall of intake
3-day diet recall	Self-administered, no interviewer required, no recall bias	Large burden to patient, literacy and motivation, possible underreporting
Food frequency questionnaire	Cost-effective, assess usual dietary intake (used most widely in research)	Uses closed ended questionnaire, low accuracy d/t recall bias, large burden to patient
Application	Detail intake data, in interview required, no recall bias	Literacy, requirement of a device or computer, requires data be reviewed by provider

etables. This step helps start lifestyle interventions related to current eating patterns. For example, a patient eats 10 times a week at fast-food restaurants for convenience with Coca-Cola, sandwich, and fries. The patient agrees this is something he would like to reduce so a goal is created to decrease this by 50% in the next 7 days and will pack a lunch on those days. You could also look at large portions versus a serving, sugar sweetened beverages, energy dense foods, and late-night eating. During the next week you give the patient a handout to review about various eating plans. Let's review the different eating plans and patterns (Table 8.2). You will notice that the majority identify proposed benefits. This is stated this way due to the fact that many of the eating plans have small studies to base the benefits on or were done over short periods of time. Few studies on eating plans are large randomized controlled trials.

TABLE 8.2 Eating plan overview

Plan	Requirements	Benefits
Low fat	15–20% fat intake	Weight loss Improved metabolic markers Improved BP Reduce all cause premature mortality
Low carbohydrate	20–60 g of carbohydrates depending on plan Protein between 1.2 and 1.6 g/kg/day	Weight loss Improved metabolic markers Improved insulin sensitivity Decreased triglycerides
Mediterranean	Whole food Point program over a week based on nonspecific dietary components	Improvement in existing heart disease Anti-inflammatory Protection against neurocognitive decline Decrease in all cause of death
Whole food plant based	Plant-based foods with minimal processing, high in fiber Avoid animal products Avoid highly refined grains, processed foods, added sugars, and oils	Improved metabolic markers Improved BP Reduction in all-cause mortality Decrease in visceral adipose tissue
Fasting	Varies from concentrated timed feeding (8 hours eating, 16 hours fasting) up to 72 hours of fasting. May also be 25% of caloric needs on several days a week	Decreased inflammation Decreased visceral adipose tissue Improved BP and metabolic and lipid profile

TABLE 8.2 (continued)

Plan	Requirements	Benefits
LCD/VLCD	Primarily meal replacement plans Calories vary from 800 to 1600 calories a day	Helpful for patients with difficulty in making food choices by removing those choices Assist in learning serving and portion control Short-term weight loss

Eating Plans and Patterns

Macronutrient

Low Fat

The normal American Diet is 35–40% of total calories from fat. Low fat is probably the one that has been around the longest. The proposed benefits include weight-loss, improved metabolic markers, improve blood pressure, and may reduce premature all-cause mortality. A low-fat eating plan has a fat intake at 15–20% of total calories. An example is the DASH diet: individuals with hypertension who were fully adherent to DASH could have prevented an estimated 400,000 cardiovascular events over 10 years. The initial DASH trial was a randomized controlled feeding study. DASH was particularly effective for those with hypertension and among black individuals. Systolic blood pressure and diastolic blood pressure demonstrated a mean decrease of 6.8 and 3.7 mmHg, respectively [6].

Low Carbohydrate

The proposed benefits include improving metabolic markers like decreased insulin levels, insulin sensitivity, increased HDL, and decreased triglycerides. Patients report improved satiety. The hypothesis is that decreased carbohydrates cause the body to burn stored fat for energy.

Low-carb eating plans include a daily limit of 20–60 g of carbohydrates depending on the plan. There's no limit on fats, but most low-carb eating plans recommend limited saturated and no *trans* fats. Protein is recommended between 1.2 and 1.6 g of protein/kg/day. The carbohydrates insulin model (CIM) of obesity theorizes that diets high in carbohydrates increase adipose tissue due to the propensity to elevate insulin secretion. Insulin directs the partitioning of energy toward storage as fat in adipose tissue. In response, hunger and appetite increase and metabolism is suppressed. Hall and associates [7] studied individuals in the lab and were not able to demonstrate the theory behind the CIM. The author, based on clinical practice, does expect that using lower carbohydrate diets in free living subjects is likely to lead to weight loss and body fat loss over the short-term when people are successful with eating changes and in clinical practice has seen this occur. Anecdotally, many providers find low carbohydrate eating plans sustainable by patients over long periods of time.

Let's move away from macronutrients to meal patterns.

Meal Plans

Mediterranean

The Mediterranean eating plan has the proposed benefits of improving heart disease, anti-inflammatory, protection against neurocognitive decline, and in all cause of death including cancer. The evidence is from the Lyon's heart study which showed a 50–70% reduction in secondary cardiovascular events [8]. The Predimed study had 7447 individuals and showed cardiovascular risk reduced by 30% even without caloric reduction [9]. Unfortunately, with the Predimed study there was a recent retraction of study results due to the way some patients were not randomized. The authors contend basic findings are the same, perhaps with a bit less enthusiasm. For treating obesity, it is important to note that the original study did not have weight loss as an outcome for

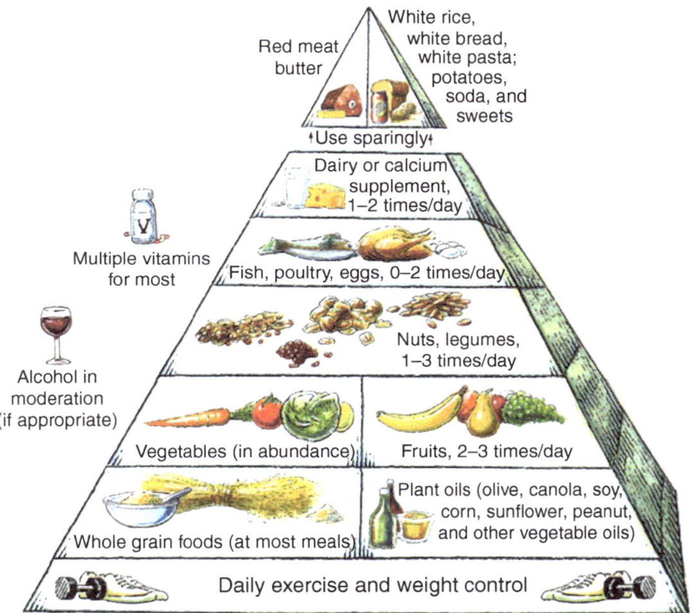

FIGURE 8.1 Mediterranean pyramid

evaluation. It seems clear from looking at the evidence the Mediterranean eating plan is a healthy eating plan and likely helps prevent some of the world's leading chronic diseases. The nutritional guidelines of the Mediterranean eating plan include nine dietary components. There's a score of 0–9 depending on the amounts consumed (Fig. 8.1). What the Mediterranean eating plan does not have in it are any sugar sweetened beverages, added sugars, processed meat, refined grains, refined oils, and other highly processed foods.

Whole Foods Plant Based (WFPB)

The proposed benefits of WFPB are improved metabolic markers, improvement in blood pressure, and reduction in all-cause mortality, while also decreasing visceral adipose tissue [10]. Multiple potential mechanisms underlie the benefits of a plant-based diet and include decreasing insulin resistance, likely due to increases in fiber and phytonutrients, food microbiome interactions, and decrease in saturated fat. Plant-based diets are also high in fiber, antioxidants, and magnesium. All of these have been shown to promote insulin sensitivity [10]. Antioxidants such as polyphenols may inhibit glucose absorption, stimulate insulin secretion, reduce hepatic glucose output, and enhance glucose uptake. WFPB is high in dietary fiber which has been linked to decrease markers of inflammation, another way to reduce insulin resistance. Finally, an eating plan high in plant-based foods and low in animal products is likely to exert beneficial metabolic effects by promoting a beneficial change in the gut microbiota profile [11]. The nutrition of this eating plan is fairly simple with avoidance of animal products, highly refined grains, highly processed foods, added sugars, and oils. There is no calorie counting as the stress is on whole foods such as legumes, leafy greens, cruciferous vegetables, starchy vegetables, whole grains, and fruits.

Meal Patterning

Fasting

The proposed benefits by proponents of fasting are decreased inflammatory markers, visceral adipose tissue, and blood pressure with improved metabolic and lipid profile. Nutrition varies from 24 hours fasting with only water to decreased caloric intake on alternate days: 0–25% of caloric needs, or 500–750 calories. Varady and colleagues [12] published short-term modified alternate day fasting: with 16 participants in an 8-week trial. The results for weight loss were 5.6 kg, and a decrease in total and LDL cholesterol was seen by 21% and 25%. The concerns were whether or not adherence over long term to the eating plan could be done or if there is sustained weight loss. There are also concentrated timed fasting, intermittent fasting with 8 hours of eating and 16 hours of fasting.

Energy Focused

Two of the most widely investigated dietary prescriptions for weight loss are low calorie diet (LCD) and very low calorie diet (VLCD). LCD nutrition includes 800–1600 kcal/day. The structure can be varied with the use of meal replacement plans for patients with obesity. This can be full or partial meal replacement plan. A full replacement plan has patients buying all the food prepackaged. A partial is the patient using packaged items for two meals and snacks with prepared food for one meal.

LCD is designed to reduce calories and often accomplished with the use of meal replacements, usually beginning with liquid shakes and possibly bars. These contain a known amount of energy and macronutrient content and allows for the structure for patients on the LCD and VLCD diets. These methods of increasing structure are believed to be helpful for patients because they reduce difficulty in food choices and challenges about what to consume. In addition, meal replacements can assist in learning serving versus portion control. The LCD and VLCD often produce greater short-term weight loss as compared which traditional food.

VLCD is very structured, 0.8–1.5 g of protein per kg per day with less than 800 kcal per day. Adherence to VLCD often needs pharmacology to decrease hunger. A meta-analysis of six RCTs comparing weight-loss outcomes of the LCDs to VLCDs found that although the VLCDs produced significantly greater weight loss in the short-term, there was no difference in weight loss between the diets in long-term follow-up of greater than 1 year [13].

There are complications to be watched for in VLCD. Vitamin deficiencies, electrolyte imbalances, hair loss, skin thinning, hypothermia, and cholelithiasis have been reported. It's important to think about special situations under which VLCD can have risk to the patient. Those patients with significant renal, hepatic, psychiatric, or a history of cardiovascular disease need very close monitoring. An example is patients with Type 2

Diabetes Mellitus may need to more closely monitor their blood sugar to assure they do not have hypoglycemic episode [14]. Most experts believe that this should only be utilized under medical supervision in a comprehensive program. These eating plans can rarely be sustained for longer than 3–6 months, and in clinical practice, compliance after a few weeks is generally poor. There are patients who might benefit; patients who have trouble selecting food, meal replacements limit their selection, people who've had no success at weight loss (keep in mind that most of our patients have been very successful at weight loss, just not successful at maintenance). Because this has such rapid weight loss initially this may be a way to help start a successful journey in the treatment of obesity. Knowing that obesity is a chronic disease should call into question the use of an eating plan that is short-term, without being very clear at the beginning there must be a transition.

Which Plan for Whom?

The A to Z study demonstrated that all four eating plans evaluated had people in the group that lost weight, but some gained. I think this is the most difficult part of treatment. How to guide your patient in choices for eating plans has multiple steps. Since we know that no one plan is the best eating plan for every patient and that long-term ability to continue an eating plan must be a part of our shared decision–making, these play a role in this decision-making. There are some ideas for considering one plan over another (Table 8.3).

TABLE 8.3 Matching patient to an eating plan

Eating plan	**Benefits beyond weight loss**
Low carbohydrate	Decreased HgBA1C
Meal replacement	Removal of food choices
Mediterranean	Improvement of chronic diseases
Low fat	Hypertension improvement
Whole food plant based	Improvement of chronic diseases

Miscellaneous Issues

Fruits and Vegetables

A randomized controlled study examined the influence on weight based on the advice of increasing fruits and vegetables with no other dietary changes [15]. This is often a recommendation of primary care providers. Solely increasing fruits and vegetables did not produce weight loss [15].

Caloric Beverage

Tate [16] found that replacing caloric beverages with water or diet beverages resulted in a weight loss of 2–2.5% during a 6-month period.

Fast Food

The American Heart Association published an article that found people who consume fast food even once a week increase the risk of dying from coronary heart disease by 20% [17]. While those eating fast food 2–3 times each week increase their risk by 50%. Eating fast food two or three times a week also was found to increase the risk of developing type II diabetes by 27%. Ultraprocessed food recently was shown to increase the number of calories eaten and absorbed [18].

Protein at Breakfast

Evidence exists that breaking a fast with 30 g of protein can decrease ghrelin throughout the day thereby reducing hunger [19]. MRI scans have shown that eating protein-rich breakfast reduces the signals in the brain that controls food motivation and reward driven behavior. Eating a breakfast with protein reduces gastric emptying, possibly through increased secretions of cholecystokinin and Glucagon-like Peptide-1 [14].

National Weight Control Registry

The National Weight Control Registry was established in 1994 and has over 10,000 individuals who have lost at least 30 pounds and kept it off for 1 year or longer. Findings from the study can assist primary care providers. The findings include eating breakfast every day, watch less than 10 hours of TV per week (author's comment: this is likely screen time in today's world not just TV), regular consumption of no calorie sweetened beverages is common, five small meals a day, and eating high-fiber low processed foods [20].

Angies's Process of Guiding Patients

After I see a patient's diary, I start with modifiable changes while they look at eating plans. Some patients just use the modifiable changes and don't ever select a plan.

1. Clean up food choices by decreasing processed foods, decrease refined sugar
2. Evaluate serving versus portions
3. Begin mindful eating
4. Assure patient is tracking food and hunger (more on tracking in behavior intervention area)
5. Guide patient in selecting a starting eating plan (provide patient with an overview of each eating plan to help guide their selection or have them continue modifiable changes)
6. Begin the day with 30 g of protein

Throughout most of the healthcare industry the answer to eating plans is to have a balanced, low calorie diet with reduced portion size. This has been helpful short-term but does not seem to be associated with sustained weight loss. These are what most of the commercial weight loss programs follow. Our role is to help the patient find a sustainable plan for long-term success. This will need the behavioral components to help patients around the roadblocks or stumbles that occur.

Practice Pearls

- Determine patient's current eating to assess patterns.
- DON'T assume a patient with obesity is eating large number of calories.
- Used shared decision-making to make modifiable changes or an eating plan.
- Patient ability to adhere to a plan long term is the most critical.

References

1. Academy of Nutrition and Dietetics. Position of the Academy of Nutrition and Dietetics: interventions for the treatment of overweight and obesity in adults. J Acad Nutr Diet. 2016;116(1):129–47.
2. Wishnofsky M. Caloric equivalents of gained or lost weight. Am J Clin Nutr. 1958;6(5):542–6. https://doi.org/10.1093/ajcn/6.5.542.
3. Hall KD, Heymsfield SB, Kemnitz JW, Klein S, Schoeller DA, Speakman JR. Energy balance and its components: implications for body weight regulation. Am J Clin Nutr. 2012;95(4):989–94.
4. Food and Drug Association. Guidance for industry: guide for developing and using data bases for nutrition labeling. Docket number: FDA-2013-S-0610. 1998. https://www.fda.gov/regulatory-information/search-fda-guidance-documents/guidance-industry-guide-developing-and-using-data-bases-nutritionlabeling#chapter_IV. Accessed 11 Apr 2020.
5. Dansinger ML, Gleason JA, Griffith JL, Selker HP, Schaefer EJ. Comparison of the Atkins, Ornish, weight watchers, and zone diets for weight loss and heart disease risk reduction: a randomized trial. JAMA. 2005;293(1):43–53.
6. Steinberg DM, Bennett GG, Askew S, Tate DF. Weighing everyday matters: daily weighing improves weight loss and adoption of weight control behaviors. J Acad Nutr Diet. 2015;115(4):511–8. https://doi.org/10.1016/j.jand.2014.12.011.

7. Hall KD. A review of the carbohydrate-insulin model of obesity. Eur J Clin Nutr. 2017;71(3):323–6. https://doi.org/10.1038/ejcn.2016.260.
8. Dontas AS, Zerefos NS, Panagiotakos DB, Vlachou C, Valis DA. Mediterranean diet and prevention of coronary heart disease in the elderly. Clin Interv Aging. 2007;2(1):109–15. https://doi.org/10.2147/ciia.2007.2.1.109.
9. Estruch R, Ros E, Salas-Salvadó J, Covas M, Corella D, Arós F, PREDIMED Study Investigators, et al. Primary prevention of cardiovascular disease with a mediterranean diet supplemented with extra-virgin olive oil or nuts. N Engl J Med. 2018;378(25):e34. https://doi.org/10.1056/NEJMoa1800389.
10. McMacken M, Shah S. A plant-based diet for the prevention and treatment of type 2 diabetes. J Geriatr Cardiol. 2017;14(5):342–54. https://doi.org/10.11909/j.issn.1671-5411.2017.05.009.
11. Tosti V, Bertozzi B, Fontana L. Health benefits of the mediterranean diet: metabolic and molecular mechanisms. J Gerontol. 2018;73(3):318–26. https://doi.org/10.1093/gerona/glx227.
12. Varady K, Bhutani S, Church EC, Klempel MC. Short-term modified alternate-day fasting: a novel strategy for weight loss and cardioprotection in obese adults. Am J Clin Nutr. 2009;90:1138–43.
13. Mulholland Y, Nicokavoura E, Broom J, Rolland C. Very-low-energy diets and morbidity: a systematic review of longer-term evidence. Br J Nutr. 2012;108(5):832–51. https://doi.org/10.1017/S0007114512001924.
14. Hamdy O. Obesity. Medscape. 2018. https://emedicine.medscape.com/article/123702-overview. Accessed 10 Apr 2020.
15. Kaiser KA, Brown AW, Brown MM, Shikany JM, Mattes RD, Allison DB. Increased fruit and vegetable intake has no discernible effect on weight loss: a systematic review and meta-analysis. Am J Clin Nutr. 2014;100(2):567–76.
16. Tate DF, Turner-McGrievy G, Lyons E, Stevens J, Erickson K, Polzien K, et al. Replacing caloric beverages with water or diet beverages for weight loss in adults: main results of the Choose Healthy Options Consciously Everyday (CHOICE) randomized clinical trial. Am J Clin Nutr. 2012;95(3):555–63.
17. Benjamin EJ, Blaha MJ, Chiuve SE, Cushman M, Das SR, Deo R, American Heart Association Statistics Committee and Stroke Statistics Subcommittee, et al. Heart disease and stroke statistics-2017 update: a report from the American Heart Association.

Circulation. 2017;135(10):e146–603. https://doi.org/10.1161/CIR.0000000000000485.
18. Hall K, Ayuketah A, Brychta R, Cai H, Cassimatis T, Chen K, et al. Inpatient randomized controlled trial of ad libitum food intake. Cell Metab. 2019;30(1):67–77. https://doi.org/10.1016/j.cmet.2019.05.008.
19. Blom W, Stafleu L, Holst J, Schaafsma G, Hendriks H. Effect of a high-protein breakfast on the postprandial ghrelin response. Am J Clin Nutr. 2006;83(2):211–20.
20. The National Weight Control Registry. n.d. http://www.nwcr.ws/. Accessed 11 Apr 2020.

Chapter 9
Foundational Component of Treating Obesity: Physical Activity

> *IN ORDER FOR MAN TO SUCCEED IN LIFE, GOD PROVIDED HIM WITH TWO MEANS, EDUCATION AND PHYSICAL ACTIVITY. NOT SEPARATELY, ONE FOR THE SOUL AND THE OTHER FOR THE BODY, BUT FOR THE TWO TOGETHER.*
>
> *PLATO*

Key Reason
The second foundational component is physical activity. Activity alone is unlikely to treat obesity; however, it has great impact on the maintenance of successful long-term treatment. It is started early in treatment to make it an underpinning of the patient's treatment plan for life.

Introduction

This chapter examines the use of physical activity as part of the treatment plan for obesity. The assessments needed of patient's current activity and ability to increase activity are reviewed. An overview of different energy expenditure types is provided. The value of physical activity, both anaerobic and

A. Golden, *Treating Obesity in Primary Care*,
https://doi.org/10.1007/978-3-030-48683-9_9

aerobic, is assessed for patients with obesity as well as the value related to other chronic diseases.

Moving into the activity component it is important to understand that although physical activity may not be integral to the active phase of obesity treatment, it has been shown to have many benefits. It increases metabolic health, supports maintenance of weight loss, improves body composition, and improves insulin sensitivity to name just a few of the benefits [1].

Increased physical activity is largely ineffective as a standalone weight loss intervention. I have heard it said that you can't outrun the pizza you ate. Let's look at the rationale behind this statement. Exercise should promote negative energy balance just as does restricting calories [2]. The energy homeostasis system sees increased energy expenditure and works to increase energy intake through hunger to protect a person from weight loss. In people with obesity this system may not be functioning correctly and responds with greater increase in hunger cues.

There is some research that exercise may be able to increase brown adipose tissue (BAT). Remember that BAT is a key in thermogenesis and therefore metabolism. This could play a key role in maintenance. Exercise causes the production of irisin which causes an increase in BAT [3].

Although many have said obesity is caused by a lack of exercise (the "move more" argument), many studies show that exercise without eating changes is ineffective [4]. A recent study demonstrated physical activity has not declined since the 1980s [5]. So clearly this is not a sole answer to treatment of obesity.

Before recommending any activity there needs to be an assessment completed, starting with the patient's current physical activity. This is done by taking a history of work and leisure activity (Table 9.1). Before prescribing an activity plan consider the screening tool PARQ-7 to see if the patient needs further evaluations like from cardiology or orthopedics before any prescription for activity.

Table 9.1 Activity level examples

Activity level	Leisure	Work
Very light	Watching TV, reading books	Sitting at a computer or desk most of the day
Light activity	Walking or non-strenuous cycling or gardening approximately once a week	Sales or office work that comprises light activities—minimal walking or lifting
Moderate activity is	Walking, bicycling, or gardening more than once a week like	Cleaning, kitchen staff, delivering mail on foot or by bicycle
Heavy or active activity	Intense walking, bicycling, or sports several times a week	Heavy industrial work, construction work, or farming

The PARQ7 screening tool is looking for symptoms of heart disease or musculoskeletal issues that would impact the patient's ability to safely increase activity from the baseline. A yes answer to any question may lead to further evaluation.

A no to all seven PARQ7 questions likely tells you that your patient is cleared for low-to-moderate physical activity such as walking.

It's also important to assess mobility, balance, and gait. People with preobesity/overweight or obesity could have compromised mobility, and this could create an increase in the risk of injury (Table 9.2).

Patients with diminished mobility may benefit from physical therapy evaluation as part of the treatment team. This professional can then guide activity options such as chair-based activities, pool-based exercises, or classes designed for people with arthritis. [Author's note: Be sure that person understands obesity as a disease so that the patient is not going into a practice that could be biased or shaming in any way.]

TABLE 9.2 Assessment of mobility, gait, and balance

Mobility and gait assessment	Observation: have the patient get up from a chair, walk 10 feet, turn around, and come back to sit down. Is this done easily and quickly or does the patient require arms on the chair to get up, have a shuffling or antalgic gait?
Balance assessment	Romberg test
	Standing on one leg
	Ask about recent falls

If either of these raise concerns, then a physical therapy consult may be in order

Evaluate for other barriers to activity beyond physical capability. Not everyone has access to safe places to be physically active near their home or work. Understanding obstacles to access can help you and your patience find solutions.

- Does the patient have a safe area to exercise?
- Is there financial ability for a fitness facility or classes?

Before we look at the evidence around activity and obesity let's be clear that physical activity (aka exercise) is great for many life situations and chronic diseases. In the realm of life's not fair comes the information that exercise can only account for 10% weight loss during the active treatment of obesity. What you ask? In fact, exercise can *possibly* undermine efforts. It does this through several mechanisms:

1. Increases the hunger hormone ghrelin.
2. Metabolic compensation: decreased expenditure the rest of the day or basal metabolism slows [6].
3. Expenditure plateau: once you exercise a certain amount your body decreases other expenditures.
4. Patients often think "we can eat more if we exercise."

TABLE 9.3 Energy expenditure terms

Resting energy expenditure (REE)	Equals resting metabolic rate or RMR depends on body size, composition, and recent energy imbalance
Thermic effect of food (TEF)	Energy used in digesting and processing ingested food
Activity energy expenditure (AEE)	Rate of energy expended during activity This is the modifiable area of TEE
Non-exercise activity thermogenesis (NEAT)	Part of AEE Energy expended for everything we do that is not sleeping, eating, or intentional physical activity Higher levels increase overall energy expenditure Fidgeting, typing, possibly standing versus sitting
Total energy expenditure (TEE)	All of the above combined

Energy Expenditure

Energy expenditure has several areas to understand (Table 9.3). Let's look at each of these to see areas that we could utilize to help in the treatment of the disease of obesity.

REE is energy used when the body is at rest. This is the number of calories needed to sustain all metabolic activities. This number is best measured using indirect calorimetry (this is not a reimbursable test so is unlikely to be found in primary care clinics). For those of us in clinical practice it can be indirectly estimated using several calculations but the one used the most in obesity treatment is the Mifflin-St. Jeor equation, this equation has been found to be fairly accurate in outpatient settings to about 10% when compared to indirect calorimetry (Table 9.4) [7].

Saeidfard [8] demonstrated that people expend an additional 54 kcal per day standing versus sitting over 6 hours.

Table 9.4 Sites for Mifflin-St. Jeor based calculators

https://www.omnicalculator.com/health/bmr
http://www.nafwa.org/mifflin.php
https://globalrph.com/medcalcs/resting-metabolic-rate-rmr/

Over the long-term increasing NEAT with standing could be a potential addition for a person, especially those with a sedentary lifestyle.

The TEF is an area of great interest in understanding more about how the body handles the food we eat. Ultraprocessed food for instance requires less energy to digest [9]. This goes toward the idea that a calorie is not just a calorie. If the body has to work to digest the food, then there is a balance created that is not there with our ultraprocessed foods.

Activity and Guidelines

Increased physical activity is in all the guidelines. They all suggest 150 minutes per week of aerobic exercise during active treatment despite a lack of evidence for any significant weight loss. I think one of the reasons to start the patient on the path of increased physical activity comes from the evidence that 250–300 minutes/week is important for maintaining the weight lost during the treatment of the disease and to help prevent the relapses. In a secondary analysis of data from a study of adult women, it was reported that individuals who achieved weight loss of 10% were engaging in approximately 275 minutes of activity per week [10]. Comparison of the National Weight Control Registry shows approximately the same amount of time is spent in activity.

Physical Activity and Aerobic Exercise

Physical activity is any movement and includes work, daily chores, climbing stairs, walking from a further parking space, and increasing daily steps. Aerobic exercise is a continuous time of activity with an intensity of moderate to vigorous such as swimming, cycling, walking, rowing, running, and high impact routines. The rate of perceived exertion (RPE) is usually used to help patients recognize what is moderate. A one on the scale is very light, waking to the bathroom, versus 10 which is not being able to do one more minute of the activity [11]. The combination of changing eating and physical activity may provide slightly more weight loss in the treatment of obesity than either alone over 18 months. In the short term <3 months there was no difference between diet-only or the combined eating and physical activity [12].

Resistance Training

The positive outcome of resistance training includes improving lean mass. Resistance training is valuable in preventing the loss of muscle mass and in patients with diabetes and increased glucose uptake by muscle. Hamdy and Uwaifo [13] wrote "27% of weight loss during the active phase of treatment could be from loss of muscle." With this in mind after patients get their aerobic goals in place adding resistance training makes sense to prevent losing muscle since the goal of treatment is losing adipose tissue. The cons of resistance training are it can be time-consuming and require equipment with training to prevent injury. STRRIDE AT/RT, a randomized clinical trial, compared aerobic training to resistance training and a combination of the two to look at what is the "best" exercise during the active treatment of obesity [14]. Balancing time commitment against health benefits the authors concluded aerobic training is the primary exercise to recommend to patients. They also concluded that resistance training increases muscle and can be especially beneficial in middle-aged people with overweight or obesity.

Writing a Prescription for Physical Activity

Sports medicine and fitness literature widely accepts that people who receive a prescription are more likely to follow through. The acronym FITTE can guide the writing of the prescription to give patients detailed and measurable goals (Table 9.5) [15].

Here are some clinical examples of the types of activities you might prescribe for a patient. You want to partner with the patient to make a decision on activities but provide examples or ideas for increasing activity. Whatever you do please don't just say "move more" as if there is magic in that.

1. Patient unable to walk—start with seated exercise, arm cycling, aquatic program, PT referral.
2. Limited mobility—walking, again considered PT referral.
3. No limitations—take stairs, standing desks, desk cycles, walk further from car- engage in noncompetitive sports.
4. 10-minute walks immediately after meals versus 10 minutes a day can decrease blood sugar postprandial especially after dinner and increase insulin sensitivity [16].
5. Referral to fitness experts (be sure this expert knows the disease of obesity).

Table 9.5 FITTE exercise prescription (ACSM)

Frequency	Number of activity sessions for a given time—the idea is to work up to 3–5 times a week
Intensity	Level the activity places on the body—this is often done through HR or ability to speak—moderate intensity is preferred—increased HR but without breathlessness
Time	Number or minutes engaged in activity – first goal is to work up to 30 minutes a day: This could be 5–6 minutes engagement, 3–10 minutes engagement, or 2–15 minutes engagement
Type	Mode or activity used—virtually any activity can be used—stairs versus elevators, parking further from a door, dancing, gardening
Enjoyment	Deriving pleasure from the activity

FITTE RX: At moderate intensity walk for 10 minutes after lunch Monday, Wednesday, and Friday in the halls at work. Saturday and Sunday walk for 10 minutes after dinner in the neighborhood. This is the goal for the next 2 weeks.

Practice Pearls

- Assessing patient's physical ability and safety is the first step.
- Next assess baseline of activity, increase slowly with the goal of long term being 200–300 minutes a week.
- Write the physical activity as a prescription for the patient using FITTE.
- In my clinical practice I generally start with simple step counting. Most everyone can afford a pedometer or their phone can track steps. If they don't have a safe place or they have inclement weather, many malls allow walkers and often there are places at their work sites they can walk.
- Increase physical activity through shared decision-making so that it is *enjoyable* and the patient will have a greater chance of sticking with the plan. Listening to a book may make a walk enjoyable for someone that doesn't like walking—local libraries have online audible books so there would be no cost.

References

1. Clamp LD, Hume DJ, Lambert EV, Kroff J. Enhanced insulin sensitivity in successful, long-term weight loss maintainers compared with matched controls with no weight loss history. Nutr Diabetes. 2017;7(6):e282. https://doi.org/10.1038/nutd.2017.31.
2. Bray GA, Kim KK, Wilding JPH, World Obesity Federation. Obesity: a chronic relapsing progressive disease process. A position statement of the World Obesity Federation. Obes Rev. 2017;18(7):715–23.
3. Cronise RJ, Sinclair DA, Bremer AA. The "metabolic winter" hypothesis a cause of the current epidemics of obesity and cardiometabolic disease. Metab Syndr Relat Disord. 2014;12(7):355–61.

4. Swift DL, Johannsen NM, Lavie CJ, Earnest CP, Church TS. The role of exercise and physical activity in weight loss and maintenance. Prog Cardiovasc Dis. 2014;56(4):441–7. https://doi.org/10.1016/j.pcad.2013.09.012.
5. Wiklund P. The role of physical activity and exercise in obesity and weight management: time for critical appraisal. J Sport Health Sci. 2016;5:151–4.
6. Benton D, Young HA. Reducing calorie intake may not help you lose body weight. Perspect Psychol Sci. 2017;12(5):703–14. https://doi.org/10.1177/1745691617690878.
7. Frankenfield D, Roth-Yousey L, Compher C, The Evidence Analysis Working Group. Comparison of predictive equations for resting metabolic rate in healthy nonobese and obese adults: a systematic review. J Acad Nutr Diet. 2005;105(5):775–89.
8. Saeidifard F, Medina-Inojosa JR, Supervia M, Olson TP, Somers VK, Erwin PJ, Lopez-Jimenez F. Differences of energy expenditure while sitting versus standing: a systematic review and meta-analysis. Eur J Prev Cardiol. 2018;25(5):522–38. https://doi.org/10.1177/2047487317752186.
9. Hall K, Ayuketah A, Brychta R, Cai H, Cassimatis T, Chen K, et al. Inpatient randomized controlled trial of ad libitum food intake. Cell Metab. 2019;30(1):67–77. https://doi.org/10.1016/j.cmet.2019.05.008.
10. Jakicic J, Davis KK, Rogers RJ, King WC, Marcus MD, Helsel D, et al. Effect of wearable technology combined with a lifestyle intervention on long-term weight loss: the IDEA randomized controlled trial. JAMA. 2016;316(11):1161–71.
11. Cleveland Clinic. Rated Perceived Exertion (RPE) Scale. https://my.clevelandclinic.org/health/articles/17450-rated-perceived-exertion-rpe-scale.
12. Johns DJ, Hartmann-Boyce J, Jebb SA, Aveyard P. Behavioural weight management review group (2014). Diet or exercise interventions vs combined behavioral weight management programs: a systematic review and meta-analysis of direct comparisons. J Acad Nutr Diet. 2014;114(10):1557–68. https://doi.org/10.1016/j.jand.2014.07.005.
13. Hamdy O, Uwaifo G. Obesity. 2018. https://emedicine.medscape.com/article/123702-overview.
14. Bales CW, Hawk VH, Granville EO, Rose SB, Shields T, Bateman L, et al. Aerobic and resistance training effects on energy intake: the STRRIDE-AT/RT study. Med Sci

Sports Exerc. 2012;44(10):2033–9. https://doi.org/10.1249/MSS.0b013e318259479a.
15. Zaleski AL, Taylor BA, Panza GA, Wu Y, Pescatello LS, Thompson PD, Fernandez AB. Coming of age: considerations in the prescription of exercise for older adults. Methodist Debakey Cardiovasc J. 2016;12(2):98–104. https://doi.org/10.14797/mdcj-12-2-98.
16. Reynolds AN, Venn BJ. The timing of activity after eating affects the glycaemic response of healthy adults: a randomised controlled trial. Nutrients. 2018;10(11):1743. https://doi.org/10.3390/nu10111743.

Chapter 10
Foundational Component of Obesity Treatment: Behavioral Intervention

WHETHER YOU THINK YOU CAN, OR YOU THINK YOU CAN'T–YOU'RE RIGHT.

HENRY FORD

Key Reason
This component of obesity treatment links with eating and activity. It is really the cornerstone of treatment where we are making the difference in long-term effective treatment. You can be the person doing this or have other team members. But regardless of who does it, this is critical to helping patients recognize roadblocks and how to go around, over, or under them to keep them moving toward their goals.

Introduction

This chapter examines the third foundational component of an obesity treatment plan, the behavioral interventions. The chapter demonstrates the linking of the three foundational components of treatment. An overview of the research regarding behavioral interventions that identifies types of intensive behavioral therapy that have been effective is

A. Golden, *Treating Obesity in Primary Care*,
https://doi.org/10.1007/978-3-030-48683-9_10

completed. Behavioral intervention reviewed includes 5As, goal setting, mindfulness, tracking, and problem solving. The chapter provides resources for readily available programs to use in primary care.

What Is Behavioral Intervention?

Behavioral intervention is education, goal setting, evaluation of successes, and any difficulties (Table 10.1). The primary goal is to do problem-solving for any setbacks or struggles since the last visit. It is often referred to as intensive behavior therapy (IBT) or intensive lifestyle intervention (ILI). Three programs that provide evidence this can be accomplished in primary are the LookAhead trial [1], Diabetes Prevention Program [2], and Canadian Obesity Network [3].

First is there a problem? Are we doing ILI or IBT in primary care? Kraschnewski [4] found after reviewing 32,519 records from 1996 to 2008 that any type of counseling for weight declined for US physicians. Weight loss counseling declined from 39.9% to 29%. And reviewing the records for diets and exercise counseling this declined as well, 16.3% to 11.3%. Yes, this was specifically evaluating physician charts but I think it still shows a problem all primary care clinicians must change.

Table 10.1 Components to begin behavioral interventions

1	Education about obesity and overview of EB plan
2	Self- monitoring
3	Eating plan selection
4	Activity prescription
5	Goals of treatment and Why patient is getting treating
	5–10% weight loss to start
	Quality of life indicator of success

Research for ILI and IBT

Our treatment begins with assessing the patient's current eating and activity behavior and then working forward to making needed changes in these two through ILI.

The prime study that has helped guide the behavior component is the LookAhead study. At the end of year one the study had a demonstrated 8.6% weight loss with the ILI participants compared with a significantly smaller 0.7% in the standard care of education [5]. The LookAhead study provided the most extensive assessment of health consequences of ILI over 10 years. LookAhead had over 5100 patients with overweight or obesity *and* type II diabetes. They were randomly assigned to a usual care group of diabetes support and education or an ILI group. Besides weight loss the ILI group was superior in blood pressure, blood glucose, HgbA1C, fitness, quality-of-life, physical function, and sleep apnea, to name a few of the outcomes. Beyond the LookAhead trial, Bray and colleagues [6] found that participants who attended group sessions every other week for 1 year after losing weight maintained 13 kg of their 13.2 kg lost. Those who receive no further ILI regained 5.1 kg during that year.

Jensen (2014) showed the largest weight loss occurred when at least 14 sessions were done over 6 months. These resulted with a 7–10% loss from initial weight. Wing [7] was able to show that IBT done over 18 months prevented weight regain using monthly sessions once patient reached a goal. Armstrong [8] studied motivational interviewing (MI) and found evidence of MI being associated with a greater reduction in body mass.

The Canadian Obesity Network uses the five As framework in primary care. Findings of their study for the five A's showed patient provider communication improved, and medical assessments for obesity and plans for follow-up care increased [9]. One of the most interesting findings in their base line data was that approximately 80% of healthcare providers were not initiating a conversation about weight with appropriate patients. Another study demonstrated that just a 90-minute training and available toolkits increased the likelihood the conversation will occur with the patient. It is their opinion that a first step is asking to start a conversation and it must occur in a bias free, sensitive, and nonjudgmental manner [10].

Evidence from a systematic review and meta-analysis of randomized controlled trials found only one of the 5 As was linked to actual weight loss: arranging a follow-up visit [11]. People with a follow-up have more weight loss at 3 months following the visit. This is consistent with the notion that contact is an important element for influencing behavior change. That said, you can't really do arrange by itself as demonstrated by LookAhead and so many others.

When starting treatment of obesity with your patients consider what your practice will label behavior interventions. For instance, behavior intervention may make people think about "fault" in their behavior. I use the term intensive lifestyle intervention (ILI). Patients seem to resonate with the term intervention as part of a treatment plan. The first intervention in my practice is to start tracking what they eat and drink. I also provide a handout on the major available eating plans from VLCD to patterns like low carb, low fat, and meal patterns like WFPB, DASH, and Mediterranean.

How Often Should Behavior Interventions Occur?

Frequency often goes from weekly, to every other week, to monthly. The structure as part of primary care is to have a patient report on progress of goals, review of challenges, assist with problem-solving, set new goals, and perhaps an educational component on obesity treatment. Be sure to document all of this. I know this seems like a lot but there are several ways to accomplish this. The evidence shows between 14 and 22 visits a year.

Does Delivery Method Matter?

A question often raised by those in primary care is do we need to do this in the office face-to-face? Donnelly [12] looked at telephone delivered ILI and found about the same effectiveness as that in the office especially in the maintenance phase. However, we don't have a method to be paid for telephone contact except perhaps the use of chronic care codes (you will need to check with your biller on those issues). Montesi [13] reviewed multiple formats for delivering ILI and reported patients with obesity in programs that provided feedback did better than those receiving just education in all delivery forms, telephone, Internet, or face-to-face.

Methods for ILI

5 As and SMART Goals

We all learned the 5 As for smoking cessation. Obesity management has modified these slightly. Medicare also has a slightly different list for the 5 As; they don't use ask and end with arrange. I particularly like the arrange which is about doing follow-up visits (Table 10.2).

Goal Setting

Part of behavioral interventions is goal setting. Of the 5As, advise and agree are all about goal setting. Use the acronym SMART to advise and document agree upon goals until the next visit. Be sure to check if the patient was able to meet their SMART goal at that next visit (Table 10.3).

TABLE 10.2 5As of motivational interviewing for obesity

			Medicare
Ask	Get the patients permission to discuss their weight	See more on this in bias and stigma	Even though Medicare doesn't have Ask—still a good starting place
Assess	Determining what is contributing cause of obesity	First assure the diagnosis is correct and then asses for obesogenic medications and obesity-related complications/ comorbidities	Assess
Advise	Provide patient options for treatment	This should be done through motivational interviewing and guided by the patient, not the provider telling the patient what to do	Advise
Agree	Create a plan with the patient	Be specific and have the plan of care documented for follow-up	Agree
Assist	Help patient institute the agreed upon plan	This is the core of this component—the ILI or IBT to assist patient in keeping on track—this is where follow-up is so important	Assist
		Medicare recognized the importance of follow up and thus the reason for their fifth A	Arrange

Table 10.3 SMART goal example

S	Specific	I will decrease my fast food intake
M	Measurable	I can do this 50% or no more than five times in 1 week
A	Attainable	I will do this for the next 2 weeks
R	Realistic	I can do this by packing my lunch
T	Timely	I will track this and report at my next appointment

Table 10.4 Mindful eating strategies

1.	Take five deep breaths prior to each mea
2.	Sit down while eating
3.	Place your food unattractive plate or bowl
4.	Eat slowly and taste each bite
5.	Take small bites
6.	Honor your hunger cues, and do not fear hunger
7.	Pay attention to the satiety cues
8.	Once you begin to feel satisfied stop eating
9.	Eat without distractions: no TV, phone on airplane mode are examples
10.	Carry foods that you like with you and that support your help, in the event that you become hungry when you're away from home or where you have stored food
11.	Sip warm tea or water prior to a meal to help calm yourself as well as to drink the eight else's that might help increase the sense of fullness

Mindfulness

Mindfulness is a method to help patients be aware of what they are eating and why (Table 10.4). Are they hungry? Eating socially? Eating for an emotion? It is important to teach this and for patients to be nonjudgmental toward themselves. Encourage them to see it as an opportunity to be more aware of how they are using food. Mindful eating can promote self-regulation that adapts over time. Daubenmier [14] published the effects of a mindfulness-based weight-loss intervention in adults with obesity. This was a randomized clinical trial. Their results showed that mindfulness led to 5.4 kg weight loss over 18 months, as well as decrease in triglycerides, fasting glucose, c-reactive proteins, and HOMA-IR. Using mindfulness in relation to eating must promote respect of the person while being in the moment with eating. This can really help patients become more aware of physical hunger and satiety to guide eating choices. I use a handout on mindful eating with strategies adapted from the Obesity Action Coalition.

Tracking

Before we're done with behavioral interventions let's look at tracking. Tracking is behavior monitoring. Intake can be tracked with apps, paper or a bite counter. Activity is generally tracked through worn devices but can be done on paper. The advantages include helping with self-efficacy and reinforcement of goal attainment. Turner-McGrievy [15] study demonstrated that physical activity app users did more intentional activity and had lower BMI at 6 months than those without monitoring. Eating monitoring did not differ in weight between paper, app, or website; however, app users were consuming less at the six-month point.

Another tracking tool is weighing at home. The National Weight Control Registry shows that 75% of people weigh themselves at least once weekly [16]. Steinberg [17] studied weighing and found daily weighing improves weight loss and adoption of weight control behaviors. Individuals who weighed everyday achieved weight loss that was significantly greater than among those weighing less than daily.

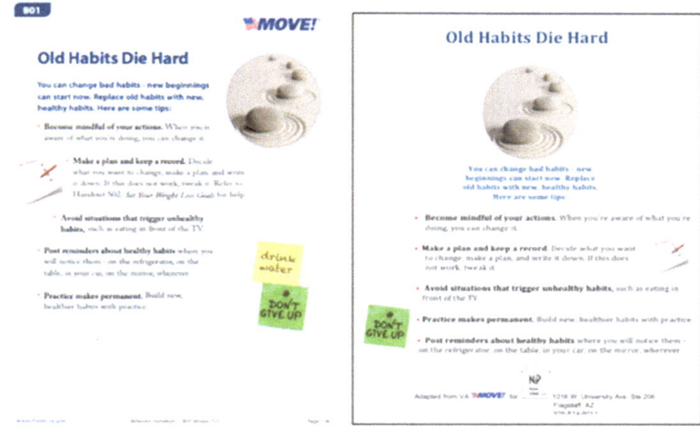

FIGURE 10.1 Example of VA Move and NP from Home Handouts

Readily Available Educational Resources

There is no reason to reinvent the wheel. There are multiple behavior intervention programs that are already packaged for educational pieces to use in your practice. An example is the VA Move program and an example of how that document has been adapted is in Fig. 10.1 VA MOVE handouts.

The diabetes prevention program also has examples; module nine of that program has a handout on managing stress. AANP has a flipchart that is a pdf and can be printed or placed on a tablet to support your teaching. This can all be utilized in your practice (see links in resources).

Problem-Solving and Goal Setting

Problem-solving is really what we can do to help patients on their journey. Helping patients set goals, teaching stress management, mindfulness, and portion versus serving size are examples of problem-solving issues. Determining if patient is finding difficulties and helping them find solutions to any difficulties following their eating and activity plan.

Goal setting needs rewards, but they should be nonfood rewards. For much of our patients lives food has been a reward if not THE reward. It's also critical to be sure that the patient and provider have an agreement on goals. An example of this is that as healthcare providers we know the benefit of 5–10% total body weight loss is a very effective goal for changing obesity-related complications; however, very few patients come into treatment with this as their goal. Frequently it can help to use outcomes besides weight as part of long-term goal setting. Ask the patient WHY they are there for treatment. When they say to lose weight, kindly challenge them. How will losing weight change something? A patient example was a lady who wanted to be able to play with her grandchildren on the floor where they liked playing. The girth of her abdomen caused her to feel short of breath and it was very difficult to get back up from being on the floor. So that was made as a long-term quality of life goal. Examples that might also be useful are lessening the impact of Obesity Related Complications (ORC), decrease in hypertension and possible lessening of medications for that ORC.

One of the barriers of doing behavioral interventions/modifications is seen by providers as being very time-consuming [18]. Many programs like the LookAhead trial, the Diabetes Prevention Program, and the five As of the Canadian Obesity Network demonstrate that this can be done in primary care. And not every piece of it has to be done by the NP, PA, or physician. It is important to look at other team members as possibilities for your intensive lifestyle intervention program. If your practice employs a registered nurse, dietitian, physical therapist, certified diabetic educator (CDE), or pharmacologist, utilize that expertise during this component of treatment. Any of these team members may be able to assist with the ILI with patients. If your practice does not employ these professionals look at your community resources. For instance many registered nurses that are CDEs have their own consulting firms. Also look for professionals holding the Board-Certified Specialist Obesity and Weight

Management (CSOWM). This test and certification confirm their understanding of obesity as a disease.

Create your interdisciplinary team or go for it alone. My practice is just me, both in primary care and my obesity practice. I do the ILI program with my patients and find it satisfying and productive.

Practice Pearls

- Behavioral modification is a cornerstone of treatment that creates long-term success.
- Resources are readily available to use in your practice.
- ILI on frequent basis is the most successful. They do not have to be hour long classes, 10–15 minutes will create success.

References

1. Look AHEAD Research Group, Wadden TA, West DS, Delahanty L, Jakicic J, Rejeski J, et al. The Look AHEAD study: a description of the lifestyle intervention and the evidence supporting it. Obesity. 2006;14(5):737–52. https://doi.org/10.1038/oby.2006.84.
2. Center for Disease Control and Prevention. National diabetes prevention program. 2019. https://www.cdc.gov/diabetes/prevention/index.html.
3. Obesity Canada. n.d. https://obesitycanada.ca/.
4. Kraschnewski J, Sciamanna C, Stuckey H, Chuang C, Lehman E, Hwang K, Sherwood L, Nembhard H. A silent response to the obesity epidemic: decline in US physician weight counseling. Med Care. 2013;5(2):39–44. https://doi.org/10.1111/cob.12038.
5. Wadden TA, Wing RR, Neiberg RH, Clark JM, Delahanty LM, Look AHEAD Research Group, et al. Four-year weight losses in the Look AHEAD study: factors associated with long-term success. Obesity. 2011;19(10):1987–98. https://doi.org/10.1038/oby.2011.230.
6. Bray G, Heisel W, Afshin A, Jensen M, Dietz W, Long M, et al. The science of obesity management: an endocrine society scientific statement. Endocr Rev. 2018;39(2):79–132.
7. Wing RR, Tate DF, Gorin AA, Raynor HA, Fava JL. A self-regulation program for maintenance of weight loss. N Engl J Med. 2006;355:1563–71. https://doi.org/10.1056/NEJMoa061883.

8. Armstrong MJ, Mottershead TA, Ronksley PE, Sigal RJ, Campbell TS, Hemmelgarn BR. Motivational interviewing to improve weight loss in overweight and/or obese patients: a systematic review and meta-analysis of randomized controlled trials. Obes Rev. 2011;12(9):709–23. https://doi.org/10.1111/j.1467-789X.2011.00892.x.
9. Vallis M, Piccinini-Vallis H, Sharma AM, Freedhoff Y. Modified 5 as: minimal intervention for obesity counseling in primary care. Can Fam Physician. 2013;59(1):27–31.
10. Rueda C, Benterud E, Bond T, Olszowka R, Vallis M, Sharma A. Effect of implementing the 5As of obesity management framework on provider–patient interactions in primary care. Clin Obes. 2013;4:39–44.
11. Alexander SC, Cox ME, Boling Turer CL, Lyna P, Østbye T, Tulsky JA, et al. Do the five A's work when physicians counsel about weight loss? Fam Med. 2011;43(3):179–84.
12. Donnelly J, Smith B, Dunn L, Mayo M, Jacobsen D, Stewart E, et al. Comparison of a phone vs clinic approach to achieve 10% weight loss. Int J Obes (Lond). 2007;31:1270–6.
13. Montesi L, El Ghoch M, Brodosi L, Calugi S, Marchesini G, Dalle GR. Long-term weight loss maintenance for obesity: a multidisciplinary approach. Diabetes Metab Syndr Obes Target Ther. 2016;9:37–46. https://doi.org/10.2147/DMSO.S89836.
14. Daubenmier J, Moran P, Kristeller J, Acree M, Bacchetti P, Kemeny M, et al. Effects of a mindfulness-based weight loss intervention in adults with obesity: a randomized clinical trial. Obesity. 2016;24(4):794–804. https://doi.org/10.1002/oby.21396.
15. Turner-McGrievy G, Beets M, Moore J, Kaczynski A, BarrAnderson D, Tate D. Comparison of traditional versus mobile app self-monitoring of physical activity and dietary intake among overweight adults participating in an mHealth weight loss program. J Am Med Inform Assoc. 2013;20(3):513–8. https://doi.org/10.1136/amiajnl-2012-001510.
16. The National Weight Control Registry. n.d. http://www.nwcr.ws/. Accessed 11 Apr 2020.
17. Steinberg DM, Bennett GG, Askew S, Tate DF. Weighing everyday matters: daily weighing improves weight loss and adoption of weight control behaviors. J Acad Nutr Diet. 2015;115(4):511–8. https://doi.org/10.1016/j.jand.2014.12.011.
18. Hamdy O. Obesity. Medscape. 2018. https://emedicine.medscape.com/article/123702-overview. Accessed 10 Apr 2020.

Chapter 11
Supportive Component of Treatment: Medications for Treating Obesity

PUT YOUR EAR DOWN NEXT TO YOUR SOUL AND LISTEN HARD.

ANNE SEXTON

Key Reason
As discussed previously the guidelines recommend comprehensive lifestyle intervention as the cornerstone of the three components in clinical practice. Research shows us that the majority of patients have had five or more concerted attempts at self-treatment prior to seeking assistance from a healthcare provider [1]. We need to take this into consideration when patients agree to treatment for the chronic disease in our clinics and look at pharmacology as a support to their lifestyle interventions early in treatment.

Introduction

This chapter examines the available pharmacology for the treatment of obesity. Indications for use of medications are discussed with general considerations. A review of each of the medications includes pharmacology of medi-

A. Golden, *Treating Obesity in Primary Care*,
https://doi.org/10.1007/978-3-030-48683-9_11

cation, monitoring, and practical considerations. A method for selecting which medication for an individual patient is introduced. A brief discussion of inappropriate medication use and the future of obesity medications are considered. Studies of interest related to the medication are reviewed.

Barriers

Very few providers are using these medications in patients who meet the requirements for AOMs. Gadde [2] reports <3.5% of eligible patients receive an anti-obesity medication. Compare this to diabetes where the concern is the burden of prescription medications. Is this another form of bias in healthcare or does it perhaps come from previous medication with difficult histories? (See the end of this chapter for more information.)

An additional barrier may be cost. As we discussed in the bias chapter many employers have not opted into obesity treatment, meaning the patient will have to pay out of pocket. Brand name medication has a monthly cost based on Internet searches of $99 to $1400. So prior authorization may take more than one attempt, if it can even be covered by employer-based insurance. Yes, I do know this takes time, but it will be worth it to treat obesity and the 236 obesity associated disorders.

The final barrier I hear from patients is their providers still see obesity as a behavioral or willpower issue. If this is the belief, the idea of a long-term medication wouldn't make sense. Of course, you are reading this book so you know obesity is a chronic disease. Medication is a tool to help treat the chronic disease of obesity, like hypertension [3]. Dr. Craig Primack posted on his Facebook page on March 15, 2019, "Obesity must be reframed so we all understand obesity as a serious, chronic, relapsing, AND treatable disease."

Anti-Obesity Medications (AOMS)

Expectation

So, what can we expect from the medications currently available? AOMs support the work of the other three components. All of the medications have been labeled to be used only as part of a comprehensive lifestyle intervention with weight loss of 4–5% at 12 weeks of maximum dose as the minimum weight loss in order to continue them.

Before looking at the medications for the treatment of obesity there is a step that should occur during assessment. Look at the current medication's patients are on and see if any are obesogenic. If you find any consider if a less obesogenic or perhaps even weight neutral medication can be substituted. An example would be a patient on a beta blocker to treat hypertension could be switched to an ARB.

Who Should Be Considered for Anti-Obesity Medications?

As with every chronic disease this answer is partially determined by disease severity. A patient with stage 2 obesity should have more aggressive treatment than a patient with preobesity. You may read in various articles the patients must "fail" intensive lifestyle interventions, but almost every patient who comes to you has successfully lost weight on various diets (eating plans) and with metabolic adaptation have regained their weight. I would encourage you to see this weight history as previous lifestyle intervention treatment and therefore give medication management an early consideration. If the patient's HgbA1C was 11 we wouldn't suggest only a visit to a dietitian, you would begin medication management WITH lifestyle intervention.

Medications should be initiated after careful evaluation for risks versus benefits—just like any medication. The labels have two categories of BMI for consideration. BMI is ≥27 kg/m^2 with an obesity-related complication or BMI is ≥30 kg/m^2. With the exception of orlistat, medications indicated for obesity target appetite mechanisms (hunger and/or satiety) (Bray 2016). They promote weight loss through effects on appetite, increasing satiety, decreasing hunger, and perhaps by aiding in resisting food cues [4].

General Considerations and Pharmacologic Initiation

Pharmacologic interventions can be helpful as an adjunct therapy with lifestyle interventions. Different patients respond to different medications, so if one option does not work consider another. Discontinue medication in patients who do not respond with weight loss of at least 5% at 12 weeks (liraglutide at 3 mg is labeled with a 4% requirement at 12 weeks). That 12 weeks is once the patient has reached the maximum dose of the given medication.

However, clinically we also want to be looking at more than weight, like the improvement in cardiovascular risk markers. Dr. Bray [5] reported that a 3% weight loss, if cardiometabolic profile had improved, may be enough to warrant continuation of the medication.

Avoid in pregnancy or in women of childbearing age, unless a pregnancy prevention plan is in place. It may be wise to do a pregnancy test at baseline prior to medication starting and consider a disclosure signature.

Of the five medications that have been approved by the FDA for long-term, phentermine/topiramate combination showed the highest mean weight loss of 9.8%. Second was liraglutide at 8.0% (Table 11.1).

TABLE 11.1 Long-term efficacy for (anti)-obesity medications

Therapy	Length of trial	Total weight loss	Mean weight loss
Orlistat	≥1 year	−5.3 kg	−6.1%
Phentermine/topiramate	≥1 year	−10.2 kg	−9.8%
Bupropion/naltrexone	≥1 year	−6.1 kg	−5.4%
Liraglutide	≥1 year	−8.4 kg	−8.0%

What Are the Approved Agents Today?

Clinically relevant information will be provided below for the medications currently available.

Short-Term Anti-Obesity Medications

Four agents are available in the United States for short-term (8–12 weeks) treatment of obesity: diethylpropion, phendimetrazine, benzphetamine, and phentermine. However, phentermine is the most used and the only short-term medication to be reviewed in this chapter.

NAME: phentermine

OVERVIEW: Phentermine has been around in the USA since 1968. It is a schedule IV medication (US, DEA).

MONITORING: Monitoring through therapy includes screening BP and HR at baseline, periodically, and after discontinuation.

PRACTICAL CONSIDERATIONS:

- Be sure to check your state board limitations. Some states limit the use of phentermine or other scheduled AOMS. Other states limit which provider type can prescribe the medication.
- Document for long-term dosing. Think about the chronicity of this disease before prescribing for only short term.

- The Endocrine Society does provide guidance on use of long-term phentermine [4]. They suggest that this can be appropriate for patients who have no cardiovascular disease, no psychiatric or substance abuse history, has been informed about therapies that are approved for long-term use, provider documents off label use in the patient's medical record, and with documentation of no clinically significant increase in pulse or blood pressure. As with any anti-obesity medication the patient must demonstrate significant weight loss (5% at 12 weeks) with phentermine. The starting dose of 7.5–15 mg per day with dose increase only if the patient is not achieving significant weight loss. The Endocrine Society guideline recommends at least monthly visits during dose escalation.
- I often use phentermine short term to assist patients with decreasing hunger while prior authorization is completed for another AOM.

Long-Term Anti-Obesity Medications

NAME: Orlistat

OVERVIEW: Orlistat is the only AOM available in OTC and prescription dosing. It was introduced in the USA as over the counter in 2006. Studies showed it decreases blood pressure, total cholesterol, LDL-C, and fasting glucose.

MONITORING: Monitoring Vitamin D levels is recommended. Patients with obesity often already have a decreased Vitamin D level as it is sequestered in adipose tissue. Discuss with patients what to do for right upper quadrant pain due to rare but possible cholelithiasis. And any patient with a history of gout should be monitored for increased occurrence.

PRACTICAL CONSIDERATIONS:

- Consider the timing of fat-soluble vitamin 1 hour before or 2 hours after taking orlistat.
- Recommendation is to limit fat intake to 30% of calories per meal.

- Some patients will find their maximum of 15 g of fat per meal to reduce side effects.
- Assure you have counseled on the risk of GI adverse events.
- Patients should understand that this is not to be taken three times a day but instead UP TO three times a day WITH meals. So if they miss a meal, they would not take the orlistat.

NAME: Phentermine/Topiramate ER

OVERVIEW: Phentermine/Topiramate ER came onto the market in 2012. This is a combination of two medications one used for years for obesity treatment and the other for things like seizure disorders and migraine prophylaxis. The combination was shown to have weight loss outcomes. There is evidence of improved cardiometabolic markers and reduction of progression to type II diabetes. This combination medication may alter oral contraceptives causing irregular menstrual bleeding; however, there was no increase in pregnancy noted.

MONITORING: Assure you have a PHQ9 questionnaire completed prior to starting medication and then monitor at times throughout the treatment for depression. Due to the phentermine, evaluate the patient for any cardiovascular risks including, but not limited to, palpitations and tachycardias. Patients you have any concerns about their cardiovascular health will need a cardiovascular evaluation at baseline which may include an EKG or referral to cardiology. Assure patients know the signs of hypokalemia as this can occur during therapy. Some patients may have an increase in heart rate so monitor throughout therapy.

PRACTICAL CONSIDERATIONS:

- Titration of dose on initiation and discontinuation with a minimum of 1 week at each dose.
- It is a Schedule IV medication.
- REMS program that needs to be reviewed prior to prescribing due to the topiramate that can cause congenital malfor-

mations (https://www.accessdata.fda.gov/scripts/cder/rems/index.cfm?event=IndvRemsDetails.page&REMS=45).

- Council the patient about the risks for mood disorders, and suicidal thoughts.
- Educate patient about avoiding alcohol as there could be an increase in sleepiness or dizziness.
- Patients must have a pregnancy prevention plan in place. Pregnancy test prior to initiation for women of childbearing age and occasionally during therapy.

NAME: Liraglutide

OVERVIEW: Liraglutide is a GLP-1 analog which stimulates glucose-dependent insulin secretion. It was approved for treatment of obesity in 2014 at a dose of 3 mg. This is in contrast to the same molecule used for diabetes management which has a dose up to 1.8 mg.

MONITORING: Blood glucose needs to be monitored closely as there is a risk of hypoglycemia when used with antidiabetic medications, especially an insulin secretagogue. Monitor BS at the start of therapy and during therapy to determine if anti-diabetic medications need to be adjusted. Liraglutide may increase heart rate; monitor resting heart rate at initiation of therapy and educate patients to report palpitations or tachycardia. Acute gallbladder issues can occur with rapid weight loss, as we know, but the incidence was higher with liraglutide. Be sure your education has included the signs and symptoms and for the patient to report to you or go to ER if abdominal pain is severe. Due to the risk of thyroid C-Cell tumors (found only in rodents) a patient found to have thyroid nodules should likely have further evaluation, neck imaging, before starting liraglutide. Counsel patients to report hoarseness or lumps in their throat. There have been reports of acute pancreatitis, again as part of your education be sure patients are aware of the symptoms (pain radiating to the back, persistent severe abdominal pain, with or without nausea and vomiting) and understand they should go to the ER. Assure adequate renal functioning before starting liraglutide, and if patient has renal impairment, be cautious while escalating doses to prevent worsening of chronic renal failure or acute renal failure. A PHQ9 should be completed prior to initiation and monitored throughout therapy for the emergence or worsening of depression, suicidal thoughts or behavior. Finally, liraglutide can cause an increase in lipase, and there is no recommendation to monitor during therapy.

PRACTICAL CONSIDERATIONS:

- This is an injectable medication so it will require patient education at your office.
- In my clinical practice titration takes much longer than the label due to the side effect of nausea. I start the medication at the 0.6 mg but if the patient cannot tolerate the nausea, then I will decrease to 5 clicks (or 0.3 mg) and increase by 5 clicks. I have the patient stay at that dose until nausea is gone and then do the next increase.
- Nausea has been the most common cause of problems and can be treated with small frequent meals. I have also used peppermint essential oil by inhalation (not ingestion) and ginger root chews. Both have been effective for my patients, and rarely is nausea a long-term issue.
- Effect on diabetes due to mechanism of action requires monitoring.
- In my clinical experience patients experience fewer cravings for sweets and carbohydrates.

NAME: Naltrexone/Bupropion ER

OVERVIEW: naltrexone/bupropion ER was approved in 2015. The combination of naltrexone and bupropion leads to much greater weight loss than either agent alone. We've used both of these medications in the past for other reasons. Studies show improvement in cardiometabolic parameters, lessened cravings, and lowered HgBA1C in patients with type II diabetes.

MONITORING: Can increase blood pressure, so BP should be monitored during initiation and with any dose escalation. PHQ9 should be monitored for increasing depression or suicidal thoughts. Patients with DM should have glucose monitored regularly.

PRACTICAL CONSIDERATIONS:

- Titration of dose on initiation and discontinuation 1 week at a time.
- Patient may not need the full bid dosing.
- Same black box warning as all antidepressants (d/t bupropion).
- Naltrexone/Bupropion ER should not be taken with a high-fat meal because of resulting significant increase in the body's exposure to both of those medications.
- There's also been reduced alcohol tolerance reported, so all alcohol intake needs to be minimized.
- If patient has depression, be sure that this is monitored very closely during discontinuation as other depression treatment may need to be increased.
- False positive urine test for amphetamines has occurred.

NAME: lorcaserin

NOTE: On February 13, 2020, the FDA requested Eisai withdraw lorcaserin from the market due to a concern related to possible cancer increase. The CAMILLA-TIMI study had 12,000 patients and was a cardiovascular outcome trial, not a cancer risk study. The study demonstrated no increase in cardiovascular risk and a reduction in risk of diabetes. The *New England Journal of Medicine* article reported no difference in cancer risk. The 3 years of data demonstrated lorcaserin with a 3.59% cancer incidence and 3.50% cancer incidence in placebo. The FDA reported a 7.7% increase in individuals receiving lorcaserin and 7.1% with placebo. There was no hearing and no publication from the FDA [6, 7].

Table 11.2 reviews the medications in alphabetical order, and Table 11.3 provides studies of interest for each of the medications.

TABLE 11.2 AOM information (for complete prescribing information for any medication: https://www.accessdata.fda.gov/scripts/cder/daf/index.cfm?event=medguide.page)

Name	Pharmacology	Dosing	SE/AE	Contraindications	Drug Interactions
Liraglutide (Saxenda)	Binds and activates the GLP-1 receptor. It is stable to the effect of DDP-4 unlike endogenous GLP-1 giving it a 13-hour half-life. This regulates appetite likely in the hypothalamus. (Mehta 2017)	Requires titration starting at 0.6 mg and by the label over 5 weeks to the target dose of 3.0 mg. No age, race, or gender adjustments are necessary. This medication is not yet studied for obesity in children or adolescents. The medication is titrated up to 3 mg and 12 weeks after reaching the maximal dose the patient needs to have lost 4% to be considered effective for continued use	Most common side effects are GI side effects, nausea, vomiting, diarrhea, and constipation. Additionally, headache, dyspepsia, fatigue, dizziness, hypoglycemia, and abdominal pain. On the label an adverse effect is noted of decreased appetite, this seems a bit odd since that is the effect that the medication is being given for—satiety and decreased hunger	The contraindications are family or personal history of medullary thyroid cancer, multiple endocrine neoplasia type II, and pregnancy. Due to the post-marketing reports of acute pancreatitis I am cautious if the patient has a history of pancreatitis (this is not a label contraindication but more a precaution and the risk of acute pancreatitis is under warnings on the label). The label does say if the patient has pancreatitis confirmed the medication should be stopped and not restarted. Avoid liraglutide in patients with a history of suicide or active suicidal ideation. Hypersensitivity to liraglutide	Due to delay in gastric emptying may impact oral medications taken at the same time. Among these are medications with a narrow therapeutic index (e.g., Warfarin), dependent on concentrations (e.g., antibiotics), or that require rapid absorption (analgesics). These medications should be monitored for effect if taken while a patient is on liraglutide or if it is being discontinued. Alcohol should be avoided as it may cause hypo- or hyperglycemia in patients with diabetes

(continued)

Table 11.2 (continued)

Name	Pharmacology	Dosing	SE/AE	Contraindications	Drug Interactions
Naltrexone/ BupropionER	Bupropion is an antidepressant that possibly acts by modulating the action of norepinephrine while naltrexone is an opioid-receptor antagonist. Studies suggest the combination works on the hypothalamus to decrease food intake regulation and mesolimbic dopamine circuit reward system to reduce food cravings, although the exact mechanism not fully understood	Each tablet contains 8 mg of naltrexone and 90 mg of bupropion. During initiation the patient starts with one tablet in the morning. Then week two is a tablet in the am and one in the pm. Week three is two tablets in the am and one in the pm and finally week four is two tablets twice a day to a total dose of 32 mg naltrexone and 360 of bupropion	Common side effects include nausea, constipation, headache, dizziness, vomiting, insomnia, and dry mouth. There may be a transient increase in blood pressure. Less common but serious reactions include hepatotoxicity assure the education for patients of S/S of acute hepatitis and to stop medication and get help from your office that day or to the ER. Acute-closure glaucoma has occurred with antidepressants. Hypoglycemia with antidiabetic medications can occur especially with sulfonylureas. Activation of mania can occur if patient has bipolar disorder	Naltrexone/BupropionER is contraindicated if patients with uncontrolled hypertension, seizure disorder, anorexia or bulimia, drug or alcohol withdrawal, chronic opioid use (d/t naltrexone). It is not to be used within 14 days of a MAO-I. It should be avoided in pregnancy. All women of childbearing age must have a pregnancy prevention plan in place. And of course hypersensitivity to any of the ingredients.	Dopaminergic medications should be avoided (e.g., levodopa and amantadine), drugs that lower seizure threshold (e.g., antihistamines, baclofen, fentanyl), other medication that are metabolized by the CYP2D6 pathway (e.g., metoprolol, warfarin)

Orlistat	Orlistat is a lipase blocker in the stomach and small intestines with minimal absorption systemically	The dosing of this medication is 60 mg OTC (Ally) and by prescription it's 120 mg (Xenical). It can be taken three times a day during a meal or within 1 hour of a meal	The side effects are almost all GI. Most common are oily fecal spotting, intestinal cramps, flatus with discharge, fecal urgency, fatty oily stool, increased defecation, and fecal incontinence. All of these increase with a higher fat meal. Post-marketing reports (although rare) are increase risk of cholelithiasis, urinary oxalate, and liver injury	Chronic malabsorption syndrome, pregnancy, breastfeeding, and ongoing or acute gallbladder issues. Additionally, patient with organ transplants, pregnancy, or bulimia should not use the medication. Hypersensitivity to orlistat	Fat-soluble vitamins may not be absorbed as well (vitamins A, D, E, and K), warfarin, antiepileptic agents, levothyroxine, and cyclosporine

(continued)

TABLE 11.2 (continued)

Name	Pharmacology	Dosing	SE/AE	Contraindications	Drug Interactions
Phentermine	Phentermine acts as a sympathomimetic thereby increasing satiety	Phentermine is available in generic form and it is fairly inexpensive in doses from 8 to 37.5 mg. The label for phentermine lists 13 weeks maximum for treatment	Palpitations, tachycardia, increased BP, overstimulation, tremor, dizziness, insomnia, dysphoria, HA, dryness of mouth, diarrhea, and constipation. In clinical practice at lower doses these are less likely except for dryness of mouth	CV diagnosis (e.g., atrial fibrillation, PSVT), uncontrolled HTN, hyperthyroidism, glaucoma, drug abuse history, and MAO inhibitor in past 14 days	(not inclusive) MAOIs should be separated by 14 days to prevent hypertensive crisis. Other stimulant medications may create higher risk for hypertensive crisis or arrhythmias. SSRIs can cause elevated BP. Be careful with any diabetes medications as they could cause an increase in hypoglycemia
Phentermine/ Topiramate ER (Qsymia)	Phentermine is a short-acting sympathomimetic while topiramate is a long-acting neurostabilizer combined see decreased hunger and increased satiety	This medication has an escalation on initiation and discontinuation. It is initiated at 3.75 mg/23 mg for 2 weeks, then it could be increased to 7.5 mg/46 mg and then two more doses, 11.25/69 mg and 15/92 mg. Many patients do quite well at the 7.5/46 mg dose	Common side effects include paresthesias, dizziness, taste alterations, insomnia, constipation, dry mouth, elevated heart rate, memory, or cognitive changes (especially difficulty with word find)	Pregnancy, breastfeeding, CV diagnosis (e.g., atrial fibrillation), hyperthyroidism, glaucoma, drug abuse history, or the use of MAO inhibitors within 14 days of phentermine/topiramate. Hypersensitivity to phentermine or topiramate	This may potentiate central nervous system depressants and hypokalemic if given with nonpotassium sparing diuretics.

Table 11.3 Studies of interest

Study of interest	Results
Phentermine: Long-term Phentermine Pharmacotherapy: An Investigation for Symptoms of Dependence, Cravings, or Withdrawal, PC-II [12]	The study included 260 participants who took phentermine 37.5 mg for longer than 2 years and then abruptly withdrew the medication to determine if there was evidence of dependence, cravings or withdrawal. The study concluded that there is not any indication that phentermine has a risk of abuse or psychological dependence (addiction). Amphetamine-like withdrawal did not occur with the abrupt withdrawal of the medication even after treatment durations of up to 21 years
Orlistat: XENDOS (Xenial in the Prevention of Diabetes in Obese Subjects)	4-year double blind study with 3305 patients with BMI ≥ 30 and both normal and impaired glucose tolerance. The purpose was to determine if using orlistat could alter the progression to diabetes. The authors concluded that lifestyle changes with orlistat compared to lifestyle alone reduced the incidence of type 2 diabetes over 4 years. This difference was greater in the impaired glucose tolerance cohort. The study also confirmed a greater weight loss while using the medication [13]
Phentermine/Topiramate: Qsymia as an Adjunct to Surgical Therapy in the Superobese (yes I hate the title too)	Study testing Qsymia in patients pre- and post-bariatric surgery compared to patients previously having surgery with no medication support. Results of this pilot study demonstrated that patients supported with medication lost more than those without the medication. Experimental group had a baseline BMI of 61.2 (control 57.0) with 24 months BMI of 33.8 (42)

(continued)

TABLE 11.3 (continued)

Study of interest	Results
Liraglutide: SCALE Obesity and Prediabetes trial [14]	2254 patients with prediabetes and obesity to determine progression to diabetes. The two groups included patients with prediabetes and usual care, and those with prediabetes, usual care, and liraglutide. The study findings showed that the group with liraglutide 60% of patients had the prediabetes reversed and of those that did go on to develop diabetes it took 2–7 times longer [15]
Naltrexone/BupropionER: COR 1 (Contrave Obesity Research) and COR II	COR I 1742 participants to study the effectiveness of treatment of body weight. This was a randomized controlled study for 56 weeks. The findings demonstrated more weight loss than placebo. (Greenway, 2010). COR II enrolled 1496 participants to look at both weight and obesity-related risk factors. This study also showed greater weight loss than placebo and found improvement in cardiometabolic markers, reported quality of life, and control of eating

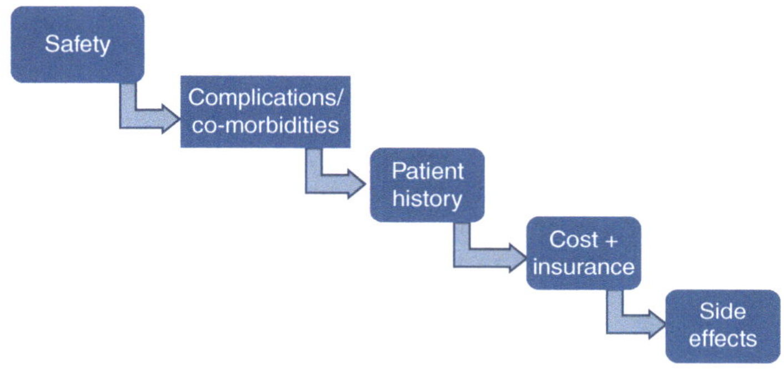

FIGURE 11.1 Five-step strategy for therapy selection

Choosing Which Medication to Start with

Here are my personal tips on choosing medication (Fig. 11.1).

Safety

As with every medication safety is first. I look at patient's history and see are there any medical issues or medications that would be a contraindication or interaction (e.g., patient has a history of seizures, so I would mark Naltrexone/ Bupropion ER (Contrave) off the list).

ORCs

Would any of the choices specifically impact the patient's complications. Are there any complications or comorbidities that can be positively affected by a particular anti-obesity medication (for instance liraglutide might be the best choice for patients with diabetes).

Pt History

Look at the patient weight history; an example is patient talking about craving sweets frequently. This may make her a likely candidate for naltrexone/bupropion or liraglutide. Another example would be a patient with depression; I might consider the AOM with bupropion, especially if the patient is not in remission (assuming there is not a reason to preclude the use of bupropion). Specifically, a patient that is on an SSRI and still has a PHQ9 score of 10 or 11 indicating mild-to-moderate depression continuing, then adding bupropion/naltrexone may provide additional benefit for the depression.

Cost

Cost has to be part of our thought process. Frequently we may find the patients insurance does not cover AOMSs. There might be a co-pay card that allows the patient to only pay $90 a month for the medication (I will digress here a minute. Can you imagine not a single medication to treat diabetes being available on a patient's insurance? I mean Really?!).

Side Effect Profile

Next step is to look at the side effect profiles. In many cases it might be something in the side effect list that the patient is not willing to even give the medication a trial. But if side effects are not a reason to help choose the medication, it's the reason that I bring patients back in 2 weeks to be sure that side effects are not an issue. An example of side effects that a patient is not willing to try would be the GI effects of orlistat. And as with all medications I always review the patient response before increasing the dose, this may be by email at 1 week if increasing a dose is recommended on that schedule.

Making a Switch

If deemed ineffective (weight loss less than 4–5% at 3 months) or if there are safety or tolerability issues at any time, guidelines recommend that the medication be discontinued and alternative medications or referral for alternative treatment approaches be considered [4]. Different patients respond to different medications; therefore, if one option doesn't work well, prescribers should consider another option.

Other Medications

Obesity specialists have found medications for other conditions that can support the treatment of obesity, although to be clear they do not have an indication for obesity treatment. Metformin improves insulin resistance found in obesity and is at least weight neutral, although some patients will have slight weight loss. Obesity does have one GLP1 that is approved for obesity (liraglutide at 3 mg), but other GLP-1s used for diabetes may also provide some weight loss, likely about 2–3%. Pramlintide has been shown to have modest weight loss for patients with obesity and DM2 [8]. Remember back to physiology, amylin regulates glucose and acts as a neuroendocrine hormone of satiety. Pramlimitide is an amylin analog and therefore may support satiety.

History of Weight Loss and Anti-Obesity Medications

The combination of fenfluramine and phentermine ("fen-phen") was used in some long-term trials with excellent results. However, fenfluramine was associated with valvular heart disease and pulmonary hypertension and it was withdrawn in 1997. In 1997, sibutramine came on to the market but was found to have cardiac adverse events and was removed in 1999. Rimonabant worked by blocking a cannabinoid receptor and was approved in 2006 in the EU but was removed in 2009 due to psychiatric adverse effects. Due to these events todays' medications all have required CV outcome studies and are aimed at impacting obesity including its complication.

What Not to Use

As we have discussed medications it is important to know what's been tried by the patient. We should also know what does not have evidence to support the use. Other medications used previously for weight loss and stopped include the following: thyroid hormone because it can cause hyperthyroidism with its attendant sequelae. A combination referred to as rainbow pills was a mixture of digitalis and diuretics causing fatal arrhythmias and electrolyte derangements. Aminorex caused pulmonary hypertension and phenylpropanolamine had incidence of increased risk of myocardial infarction and stroke.

Some agents/supplements that initially showed promise were later demonstrated to be poor prospects in rigorous randomized intervention trials. These include the following: Guar gum, Chitosan, Axokine, St. John's wort, Psyllium, Conjugated linoleic acid, Chromium, Caffeine, Ephedrine, and Ginseng [8]. The Obesity Society is also doing a literature review for many more supplements and will publish this systematic review in the upcoming year. The FDA [9] has a consumer alert about over-the-counter "Weight loss" pills. Additionally, The Obesity Society [10] provides patient pages and one is about supplements.

Future

Many pharma companies are working to find new solutions for us to use in support of patients being treated for obesity. There is so much research going on, much still in phase one or even preclinical studies (Table 11.4) [11].

TABLE 11.4 Future of AOM

Class	Activity	Examples
Gut hormones and incretin targets	Delay gastric emptying, change hormones to use peripheral signaling to the brain	New glucagon-like-peptide-1 (GLP-1) analogues (semaglutide and oral equivalents), amylin mimetics (davalintide, dual amylin and calcitonin receptor agonists), dual action GLP-1/glucagon receptor agonists (oxyntomodulin), triple agonists, peptide YY, leptin analogues (combination pramlintide-metreleptin)
Centrally acting	Acting on the brain to either increase satiety or decrease hunger	Setmelanotide, neuropeptide Y antagonist (velneperit), zonisamide-bupropion (empatic), cannabinoid-receptor antagonists
Novel targets	Various actions	Methionine aminopeptidase 2 inhibitor (beloranib), lipase inhibitor (cetilistat), triple monoamine reuptake inhibitor (tesofensine), fibroblast growth factor 21, anti-obesity vaccines

Practice Pearls

- Few patients that are eligible are receiving medication support (is this a bias?).
- Medication success is 5% weight loss at 12 weeks of maximum dose.
- Different patients respond to different medications so if one doesn't work try a different one.
- Medications are a support component to the foundational components of obesity treatment.

References

1. Kaplan LM, Golden A, Jinnett K, Kolotkin RL, Kyle TK, Look M, et al. Perceptions of barriers to effective obesity care: results from the national ACTION study. Obesity. 2016;26:61–9. https://doi.org/10.1002/oby.22054.
2. Gadde K, Apoizan J, Berthoud H. Pharmacotherapy for patients with obesity. Clin Chem. 2018;64(1):118–29. https://doi.org/10.1373/clinchem.2017.272815.
3. Heymsfield SB, Wadden TA. Mechanisms, pathophysiology and management of obesity. N Engl J Med. 2017;376(3):254–66.
4. Apovian CM, Aronne LJ, Bessesen DH, McDonnell ME, Murad MH, Pagotto U, et al. Pharmacological management of obesity: an endocrine society clinical practice guideline. J Clin Endocrinol Metab. 2015;100(2):342–62.
5. Bray G, Fruhbeck G, Ryan D, Wilding J. Management of obesity. Lancet. 2016;387(10031):1947–56.
6. Bohula EA, Phil D, Wiviott SD, McGuire DK, Inzucchi SE, Kuder J, Im K, et al. Cardiovascular safety of lorcaserin in overweight or obese patients. N Engl J Med. 2018;379:1107–17. https://doi.org/10.1056/NEJMoa1808721.
7. U.S. Food and Drug Administration. FDA requests the withdrawal of the weight-loss drug Belviq, Belviq XR (lorcaserin) from the market. 2020. https://www.fda.gov/drugs/drug-safety-and-availability/fda-requests-withdrawal-weight-loss-drug-belviq-belviq-xr-lorcaserin-market. Accessed 12 Apr 2020.
8. Hamdy O. Obesity. Medscape. 2018. https://emedicine.medscape.com/article/123702-overview. Accessed 10 Apr 2020.
9. U.S. Food and Drug Administration. Beware of products promising miracle weight loss. 2015. https://www.fda.gov/consumers/consumer-updates/beware-products-promising-miracleweight-loss. The Obesity Society (n.d.) provides patient pages and one is about supplements.
10. Srivastava G, Apovian C. Future pharmacotherapy for obesity: new anti-obesity drugs on the horizon. Curr Obes Rep. 2018;7(2):147–61. https://doi.org/10.1007/s13679-018-0300-4.
11. Hendricks M, Istratiy Y, Greenway F. Addiction potential of phentermine prescribed during long-term treatment of obesity. Int J Obes (Lond). 2014;38:292–8.
12. Torgerson J, Hauptman J, Boldrin M, Sjöström L. XENical in the Prevention of Diabetes in Obese Subjects (XENDOS) study: a randomized study of orlistat as an adjunct to lifestyle changes

for the prevention of type 2 diabetes in obese patients. Diabetes Care. 2004;27:155–61.

13. NIH Clinical. Trials.gov. 2019. Qsymia as an adjunct to surgical therapy in the superobese. https://clinicaltrials.gov/ct2/show/NCT02301416.
14. Le Roux C, Astrup A, Fujioka K, Greenway F, Lau D, Gaal L, et al. 3 years of liraglutide versus placebo for type 2 diabetes risk reduction and weight management in individuals with prediabetes: a randomised, double-blind trial. Lancet. 2014;389(10077):1399–409.
15. Apovian C, Aronne L, Rubino D, Still C, Wyatt H, Burns C, Kim D, COR-II Study Group, et al. A randomized, phase 3 trial of naltrexone SR/bupropion SR on weight and obesity-related risk factors (COR-II). Obesity. 2013;21(5):935–43. https://doi.org/10.1002/oby.20309.

Chapter 12
Supportive Component of Treatment: Procedures and Surgery

WE ARE KEPT FROM OUT GOAL, NOT BY OBSTABLES BUT BY A CLEAR PATH TO A LESSER GOAL.

ROBERT BRAULT

Key Reason
Procedures and surgeries should be considered for all patients that meet the eligibility requirements. American Society for Metabolic and Bariatric Surgery [1] reports that only about 1% of patients eligible for bariatric surgery are receiving this care. It is critical for primary care providers to understand appropriate referrals for procedures and surgery for patients with obesity.

Introduction

This chapter examines specific procedures and surgeries currently available to patients. The criteria for patient selection are also included. The primary care provider role is reviewed from referral to preparation to the aftercare that is lifelong for patients with obesity that have had surgery.

A. Golden, *Treating Obesity in Primary Care*,
https://doi.org/10.1007/978-3-030-48683-9_12

TABLE 12.1 Contraindications and items not contraindicated to bariatric surgery

Contraindications to bariatric surgery	Active substance abuse
	Active psychiatric disease
	Active binging/bulimia
	Noncompliance
	Poor competence
NOT contraindications to bariatric surgery	HgbA1c > 8%
	Age
	New Cancer diagnosis

Bariatric surgery and procedures are treatment options for patients with obesity. There are devices and surgeries that can benefit the patient in their obesity treatment. Surgery is a risk strategy; the more severe the disease, the more important it is for discussion on a referral to a bariatric surgery program occur early in treatment. There are patients where bariatric surgery is contraindicated (see Table 12.1).

Current criteria for bariatric surgery:

- BMI ≥ 40 kg/m^2 providing surgical risk is acceptable.
- BMI ≥ 35 kg/m^2 with one obesity related disease.
- BMI of 30–34.9 kg/m^2 if the patient has type II diabetes or metabolic syndrome.
- An inability to achieve and maintain weight loss with prior weight loss efforts.

How Bariatric Surgery Works

For years bariatric surgery was thought to be successful related to weight loss due to malabsorption and/or restrictions. In fact, the evidence now demonstrates changes in the microbiome, decrease in hunger hormones, and increase in satiety hormones is the actual outcome from the surgery.

TABLE 12.2 Obesity-related complication and expected resolution

ORC	Resolution percent
Sleep apnea	73–98%
GERD	92–98%
Hyperlipidemia	63%
HTN	52–98%
DM	78–83%
NAFLD	90%
Degenerative Joint Disease	41–76%
Quality of Life	95% improved
Mortality	40–89% reduction

Refs. [3, 4]

Additionally, surgery is impacting the obesity-related complications through the improvement in obesity (Table 12.2).

Surgery

Today's bariatric surgery procedures are Roux-en-Y gastric bypass, vertical sleeve gastrectomy, laparoscopic adjustable gastric banding, and biliopancreatic diversion with duodenal switch (see Fig. 12.1).

The most common surgery being done in the USA is a sleeve gastrectomy. The Roux-en-Y gastric bypass is now the second most common [2]. Research on patients post-surgery demonstrates the change in metabolic profiles with increase in postprandial circulating GLP-1 and PYY levels [6]. The remission of Type 2 Diabetes occurs almost immediately after surgery and before weight loss occurs.

Patients report being less hungry even in the presence of decreased food amounts—this suggests that bariatric procedures suppress appetite even with reduced energy stores which usually stimulate food intake. Among possible mechanisms with the two most common surgeries is an alteration of appe-

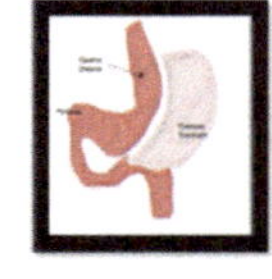
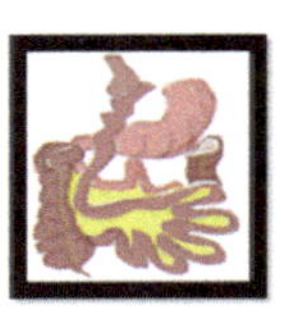
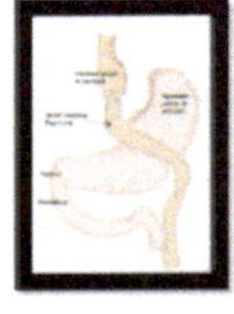

FIGURE 12.1 Common bariatric procedures approved by ASMBS [5]

tite due to a change in the communication between the GI tract and the brain. This is often referred to as the "gut brain axis" and an area of research at this time. The point here is that we cannot attribute the effect of bariatric surgery simply to mechanical alterations of the capacity of the stomach for food or the decrease in absorption of nutrients. The surgeries appear to lower the body defense of the adipose tissue mass meaning the body will allow fat mass decrease to occur. The theory is this effect on the gut-brain axis impacts satiety and hunger as well as a change in the homeostatic regulation [7].

The two main surgeries do indeed decrease the size of the stomach. Roux-en-Y gastric bypass creates a small pouch that is attached to the jejunum. Ninety-five percent of food then bypasses the stomach and duodenum. The vertical sleeve removes 70% of the stomach causing an acceleration of gastric emptying. But as mentioned this is not the whole story. There is a complex mechanism with ongoing research [8].

Mortality rate for the surgeries makes them very safe. The Roux-en-Y gastric bypass and the vertical sleeve gastrectomy are at 0.2–0.3%. One other thing of note is that the patients with a gastric band or Roux-en-Y are likely to require surgical revisions at approximately the 10-year mark. One of the barriers to surgery for patients with severe disease includes the high cost which may not be covered by insurance [8]. This provides us with another avenue for advocacy.

Table 12.3 Weight loss with devices and weight loss estimates [9]

Device	TBWL	Placebo
ReShape	6.8	3.3
Obalon	6.6	3.4
Obera (open label not sham as others in studies)	10.2	6.6
VBLOC (at 18 months)	8.8%	3.8%
AspireAssist	14.2–19.8% (more for patients with higher BMI)	4.9%
Overstitch	15.6	N/A (not studied against sham device)

Devices

There are also devices that can have a role in treatment. These devices are implanted via endoscopy and are designed for the most part to mimic bariatric surgeries. The devices currently available are intragastic balloons (IGB), aspiration therapy, endoscopic sleeve gastroplasty, and vagal blocking. Devices have varied efficacy (Table 12.3) and adverse effects (Table 12.4).

Intragastic Balloons

The question may be is there a role for temporary devices to treat obesity since they are short-term devices for a long-term chronic disease? And the answer, the jury is still out, there is some data at 12-month mark for some weight loss maintenance and reduction in ORCs. The original studies of the IGB demonstrated reduction in metabolic syndrome and type 2 diabetes rates even 12 months later. Data demonstrates that 12 months after removal there is a continued maintenance of weight loss and for about one quarter of patients' mainte-

TABLE 12.4 Prevalence for adverse events with devices [9, 10]

Intragastric balloons	
Vomiting	86%
Gastric ulceration	ReShape 10%
	Orbera 0% Obalon 0.9%
GERD	Orbera 30%
AspireAssist	
Peristomal granulation	40.5%
Abdominal pain	37.8%
Skin irritation	17%
Dyspepsia	6.3%
Nausea/vomiting	17%
VBLOC	
Nausea	11%
Pain at generator site	38%
Pain, abdominal	12%
Heartburn	23%
Problems swallowing	8%
Eructation	8%

nance was holding at the 5-year mark. The FDA label for use of this system is a BMI of 30–40 kg/m^2 and participation in a medically supervised program. Safety for devices is generally good and efficacy has been better than behavior modification alone in short-term studies. The devices are removable and repeatable. Some say that they're affordable but that depends on the patient's financial situation, rarely are they covered by insurance.

Aspiration Therapy

Aspiration therapy allows the patient to remove food after eating a meal. There is an implanted tube that can be opened to allow gastric contents to be aspirated. The device reduces the food entering the small bowel and seems to also decrease the amount of food consumed. Food particles that can be aspirated are small at less than 5 mm so there in an increase need to chew food longer to reduce the particle size. The FDA label for use of this system is a BMI of 35–55 kg/m^2. Initial food intake is pureed food and a reduction in calories. The contraindications include previous gastric ulcers that did not resolve with treatment, uncontrolled BP (with medication and BP >160/100), clotting disorders, eating disorders (including bulimia, anorexia, BED, and night eating syndrome), anemia, clotting disorders, serious pulmonary or CV disease, chronic abdominal pain, pregnancy, lactation, and physical or mental disability that interfere with ability to follow instructions.

Endoscopic Sleeve Gastroplasty

Only the suturing procedure, Overstitch, is approved in the USA. Overstitch uses suturing devices along the greater curvature creating a tube shape. The mechanism thought to work with this procedure is delayed gastric emptying and increased satiety. The FDA label for use of this system is a BMI ≥ 30 kg/m^2. In a subset of patients, in the multi-center report, there were demonstrated reductions in A1C, systolic BP, and serum triglycerides [11]. The contraindications are stomach ulcers, current or history of gastric cancer, prior stomach surgery, and clotting disorders.

Vagal Blocking

VBLOC (vagal blocking devise) is approved for people 18–65 years old, with a BMI of 40–45 or >35 with an obesity-related complication. An additional requirement is that patients must have tried to lose weight in a supervised weight management program within the past 5 years. The concept is to control hunger between meals as well as signal satiety earlier with eating. The device sends pulsed electrical stimulation to the vagal nerve. There is an external clinician program to allow the therapy to be adjusted. There was sustained weight loss at 18 months. Contraindications include liver cirrhosis, portal hypertension, esophageal varices, and other implantable devices [12].

Hydrogel Matrix

Newest on the market in 2019 is Gelesis 100 which will be sold as Plenity when it becomes available in 2020. This is a hydrogel matrix of cellulose and citric acid. The capsule has nonaggregating particles that absorb water and increases in volume to fill the stomach and small intestines. Dosing of this is one capsule taken before lunch and dinner. Study showed >50% of people with at least 5% weight loss and 27% lost at least 10%. The indications are any patient with BMI >25 kg/m^2. The side effects are GI and reported as minimal. The only contraindication is listed as a caution and that is severe reflux or ulcers. There is no restriction on the length of time this can be used. This seems to be somewhere between oral medication and devices [13].

Primary Care Role

- Assessment and discussing with a patient for a possible referral.
- Potentially doing their follow-ups post-surgery due to distance to the surgery program center or if the patient has had “tourism” surgery.
  - More Americans are traveling to other countries where the surgery is cheaper than in the USA.

Lifetime Monitoring Post-Surgery

There's a great deal of monitoring for the patient's life.

- Fat-soluble vitamins, B12, D, A, E, and K.
- Thiamine, folate, iron, calcium, zinc, and in many cases copper.
- Bone density should be monitored.

As we look at the vitamins that need to be monitored, it is easy to see why anemia can occur, especially pernicious anemia. For more detailed explanation and understanding of the complete follow-up, the ASMBS has a guideline to assist [15].

Patients post-operatively long term can have weight regain. This is the same pathophysiology as with patients who have medical management of obesity, indicating the chronic relapsing nature of this disease. Patients who have had bariatric surgery need close follow-up both for the post-surgical adverse events (Table 12.5) and nutritional needs as well as follow through due to the chronic nature of the disease.

Table 12.5 Prevalence of adverse events with surgical procedures [14]

Dumping	70%
Dairy intolerance	50%
Constipation	40%
Headaches	40%
Depression	15%
Hair loss	33%
Vitamin B12 deficiency	25%
Arrhythmias	10%
Incisional hernias, anemia, diarrhea, or abdominal pain	15%
Single or multiple vitamin deficiencies not involving vitamin B12	10%

Practice Pearls

- Consider appropriate referral for surgery early and discuss with the patient.
- Understand that surgery works beyond restriction and malabsorption.
- Patients need continued monitoring post-op. Consider that we do monitoring post-CABG, why would this surgery for a chronic disease be any different?

References

1. American Society for Metabolic and Bariatric Surgery. New study finds most bariatric surgeries performed in northeast, and fewest in south where obesity rates are highest, and economics are weakest. 2018. https://asmbs.org/articles/new-study-finds-most-bariatric-surgeries-performed-innortheast-and-fewest-in-south-where-obesity-rates-are-highestand-economies-are-weakest.
2. Mattar S. Bariatric surgery: prevalence and treatment. ASMBS presentation. 2018. https://asmbs.org/app/uploads/2018/09/5-bariatric-surgery-samer-matter.pdf. Last accessed 5/12/2019.
3. Arterburn DE, Courcoulas AP. Bariatric surgery for obesity and metabolic conditions in adults. Br Med J. 2014;349:g3961. https://doi.org/10.1136/bmj.g3961.
4. Brethauer S, Chand B, Schauer P. Risks and benefits of bariatric surgery: current evidence. Cleve Clin J Med. 2006;73:1–16. https://my.clevelandclinic.org/ccf/media/files/Bariatric_Surgery/schauerbest.pdf. Accessed 12 Apr 2020.
5. Neff K, le Roux C. Bariatric surgery: a best practice article. J Clin Pathol. 2013;66:90–8.
6. De Silva A, Bloom SR. Gut hormones and appetite control: a focus on PYY and GLP-1 as therapeutic targets in obesity. Gut Liver. 2012;6(1):10–20. https://doi.org/10.5009/gnl.2012.6.1.10.
7. Schwartz M, Seeley R, Zeltser L, Drewnowski A, Ravussin E, Redman L, Leibel R. Obesity pathogenesis: an endocrine society scientific statement. Endocr Rev. 2017;38(4):267–96. https://doi.org/10.1210/er.2017-00111.
8. Heymsfield SB, Wadden TA. Mechanisms, pathophysiology and management of obesity. N Engl J Med. 2017;376(3):254–66.

9. Sullivan S. Endoscopic medical devices for primary obesity treatment in patients with diabetes. Diabetes Spectr. 2017;30(4):258–64. https://doi.org/10.2337/ds017-004.
10. Thompson C, Abu Dayyeh B, Kushner R, Sullivan S, Schorr AB, Amaro A, et al. Percutaneous gastrostomy device for the treatment of class II and class III obesity: results of a randomized controlled trial. Am J Gastroenterol. 2016;112(3):447–57. https://doi.org/10.1038/ajg.2016.500.
11. Sharaiha RZ, Kumta NA, Saumoy M, Desai AP, Sarkisian AM, Benevenuto A, et al. Endoscopic sleeve gastroplasty significantly reduces body mass index and metabolic complications in obese patients. Clin Gastroenterol Hepatol. 2016;15(4):504–10.
12. Papasavas P, Chaar M, Kothari S. American Society for Metabolic and Bariatric Surgery Clinical Issues Committee. American Society for Metabolic and Bariatric Surgery position statement on vagal blocking therapy for obesity. Surg Obes Relat Dis. 2016;12(2016):460–1.
13. Greenway FL, Aronne LJ, Raben A, Astrup A, Apovian CM, Hill JO, et al. A randomized, double-blind, placebo-controlled study of gelesis100: a novel nonsystemic oral hydrogel for weight loss. Obesity. 2019;27(2):205–16. https://doi.org/10.1002/oby.22347.
14. Hamdy, 2018 Hamdy O. Obesity. Medscape. 2018. https://emedicine.medscape.com/article/123702-overview. Accessed 10 April 2020.
15. Mechanick JI, Youdim A, Jones DB, Garvey WT, Hurley DL, McMahon M, et al. Clinical practice guidelines for the perioperative nutritional, metabolic, and nonsurgical support of the bariatric surgery patient – 2013 update: cosponsored by American Association of Clinical Endocrinologists, The Obesity Society, and American Society for Metabolic & Bariatric Society. Obesity. 2013;21(1):S1–27.

Part III
Putting It All Together in Clinic

After completing the education on obesity as a disease and the current treatment options the next step is putting this into practice. This section will provide several examples of how this can be accomplished and include billing information so that the practice can be paid for the work being done.

Chapter 13
Billing for Obesity Treatment

THE SECRET OF GETTING AHEAD IS GETTING STARTED.

MARK TWAIN

Key Reason
Treating obesity is necessary, but every practice needs to know they can be paid to treat this disease. This chapter will demonstrate the coding and documentation needed to assure that the great work being done is reimbursed.

Introduction

This chapter examines practice profiles for payment models for primary care treatment of obesity. An overview of documentation needed for commercial and government insurers is covered. The codes that may be utilized are also reported. Preventative and traditional office visits are discussed. Examples using cases are provided.

So, all this information is great isn't it. But you have heard the urban myth you can't get paid for treating obesity

A. Golden, *Treating Obesity in Primary Care*,
https://doi.org/10.1007/978-3-030-48683-9_13

by commercial insurers. Well fortunately I do, and you can. And it doesn't have to be complicated (although it can be complicated if you want to stretch your billing acumen). You already know how to code for chronic diseases and office visits. Now all that said there are still barriers with a few companies and unfortunately Medicare is the example. More on this in a bit.

The first thing we need to do is make sure that we're documenting correctly for obesity. Assure an accurate BMI. The patients need to have their height measured at least once a year, and not what is currently done in most places which is stated height. Then with every visit the weight and BMI need to be in the note. Most of our EHRs calculate the BMI so that isn't really any stretch at all.

The majority of insurers are paying for BMI greater than 30; however, if the BMI is greater than 27 with obesity-related complications I frequently code as obesity E66.8 and my documentation reflects the stage of obesity, then I do not use the BMI code. The majority of E&M coding is the same as any other office visit: 99201–99205, for new patients, and 99211–99215, for established patients. Then the ICD-10 code for obesity E66.8 is my preferred code and here is an example why. For instance, E66.1 is obesity due to excess calories. Yet many of my patients are not consuming dramatically increased calories so this would be a poor code.

Most of obesity treatment is really focused around counseling and education so you can easily bill by time. This has specific documentation which will be shown shortly. An example is a patient with the provider for 25 minutes and 15 minutes of that was spent in counseling and education. This will let you bill a 99214 even without medical complexity or meeting the requirements for history and physical that you usually think of for 99214. Greater than 50% of the time must be documented as spent in counseling. (See Fig. 13.1.)

BILLING CODES					
Outpatient–NEW PATIENT					
CODES	99201	99202	99203	99204	99205
TIME in minutes	10	20	30	45	60
Outpatient –ESTABLISH PATIENT					
CODES	99211	99212	99213	99214	99215
TIME in minutes	5	10	15	25	40

FIGURE 13.1 E&M coding by time [1]

Added Complexity

First a quick disclaimer. Once past the straightforward coding that we all do day in and day out with the required components of the history and physical and medical complexity, or time, the coding can get more complicated. I will do an overview here but recommend you sit with your organizations biller to determine compliance with the different insurance contracts you have in your practice.

Preventative Coding

In many commercial plans that have PPO type coverage (not HMO) there may be the opportunity for 12–26 preventative visits a year. This was part of the mandate in the Patient Protection Affordable Care Act. Keep in mind though the codes can be used for smoking cessation, weight counseling, alcohol counseling, etc. One nice advantage for the patient is this code is without co-pay or deductible. This also can generate more income for the provider as the preventative codes often pay about 125% more than the routine office visits.

It is important to assure the patient has any preventative benefits with their insurance. Otherwise a resubmission of the

Prevention codes		
NEW PATIENT	Age	Code
Preventive Care Initial	18-39	99385
Preventive Care Initial	40-64	99386
65 Medicare codes see other chart		
ESTABLISHED PATIENT		
Preventive Care Follow-Up (may be able to use multiple times in a year)	18-39	99395
Preventive Care Follow-Up	40-64	99396
65 Medicare codes see other chart		

FIGURE 13.2 Preventive codes [2]

bill may have to be completed. Someone in your practice may do these prior authorizations or you can have the patient check with their insurer. See Fig. 13.2 for prevention codes.

Counseling Codes

There are other codes that might be paid with an outpatient visit for counseling as well (Fig. 13.3). These codes are specifically for counseling and are done with a modifier on the billing. If using a counseling code (99401–99403), then normal E&M coding (not by time) would be used with appropriate documentation. This is an example of an outpatient office visit with counseling code. 99213 with diagnosis code E66.8, add modifier 25 or 33 and 99401 (or 99402, 99403) and Z code for BMI Z68.35 (BMI 35.2), and counseling code(s) Z71.3 (dietary surveillance and counseling), and/or Z71.89 (exercise counseling) [3, 4]. A side note, even if I am not using counseling, I often use many of the Z codes with my usual E&M codes (Fig. 13.4).

FIGURE 13.3
Counseling codes

Counseling	Time in minutes
99401	15
99402	30
99403	45
99404	60

Z Codes	
Screening	
Z13.1	Encounter for screening for diabetes mellitus
Z13.2	Encounter for metabolic and other endocrine disorders
Z13.21	Encounter for screening for nutritional disorder
Z13.29	Encounter for screening for other suspected endocrine disorder (includes screening for thyroid disorder)
Z13.228	Encounter for screening for lipoid disorders
Counseling	
Z71.89	Other specified counseling–exercise counseling
Z71.3	Dietary counseling and surveillance
Code	BMI
Z68.25	25.0-25.9
Z68.32	32.0-32.9
Z68.39	39.0-39.9
You can see a pattern, but it changes going further	
Z68.41	40.0-44.9
Z68.42	45.0-45.9
Z68.43	50.0-59.9
Z68.44	60.0-69.9

FIGURE 13.4 Z codes

Codes Specific to Obesity

There are seven common codes that are found related to obesity (Fig. 13.5). They have inherent issues with them. The first being E66.0: Obesity due to excess calories. As the dis-

ICD10 related to obesity 13.5	
E66.0	Obesity due to excess calories
E66.01	Morbid or severe obesity due to excess calories
E66.1	Drug-induced obesity
E66.2	Morbid or severe obesity with alveolar hypoventilation
E66.3	Overweight
E66.8	Obesity, Other (MY USUAL CODE)
E66.9	Obesity, unspecified

FIGURE 13.5 Obesity codes—rarely do I use a BMI with these codes as the patients have so many complications/comorbidities that I don't have space on the superbill. It is in my documentation of course

cussion related to obesity has occurred much has been learned that it is not just calories but the way those calories are utilized and the underlying energy use of the body that can impact the disease of obesity, so this is a difficult code to be assured of as correct. Many EHR's do not allow unspecified diagnosis but will go with "other" so for this reason this has become my most common ICD10 code. There is hope that the ICD11 coding system will expand on obesity diagnosis to allow providers to be more accurate.

Medicare and Obesity

Medicare does not pay for the medical management of obesity as a disease despite having acknowledged obesity as a disease. This means that if you see the patient for the medical management of obesity and code as such the claim will be denied. There is also no coverage for anti-obesity medications. Medicare will pay for surgery if the patient meets the qualifications. What Medicare does allow is up to 22 visits with no co-pay for intensive lifestyle intervention which they call intensive behavioral therapy. This includes screening for obesity in adults using the BMI and dietary assessment. Intensive behavior therapy is used to promote sustained

Intensive behavioral therapy - 5A's

Assess	Ask about behavioral risks and factors affecting choice of behavior change goals or methods
Advise	Give clear, specific, and personalized behavior change advice, including information about personal health harms and benefits
Agree	Collaboratively select appropriate treatment goals and methods based on the beneficiary's interest in, and willingness to, change behavior
Assist	Using behavior change techniques (self-help and/or counseling), aid the beneficiary in achieving agreed-upon goals by acquiring the skils, confidence and social or environmental supports for behavior change, supplemented with adjunctive medical treatments when appropriate
Arrange	Schedule follow-up contacts to provide ongoing assistance or support and to adjust the treatment plan as needed

FIGURE 13.6 Medicare 5As of IBT

weight loss with high intensity interventions on diet and exercise. You must follow the five As of IBT that have been set up by Medicare, and your charting needs to demonstrate that you did these (see Fig. 13.6) [5].

Notice that these five As don't start with the word ask, as we have seen with other methods of approaching the patient. IBT for Medicare is only for those in a Medicare fee-for-service program. This is viewed as a preventative service. This is a way for a patient to have no Medicare part B deductible for up to 22 visits. Medicare does have rules on how these visit schedules can occur, there's one *face-to-face* visit for every week for the first month, then a face-to-face visit every other week for months two through six. Medicare will only pay if the BMI is ≥ 30 kg/m^2 and will only continue after 6 months if the patient has at least a 3 kg weight loss. If they have lost 3 kg, then the final visits are once a month for the last 6 months. This is an annual renewable benefit. It is limited to outpatient and specific providers. Primary care providers are included in the providers that can provide IBT. There is specific documentation required (see documentation at the end of this chapter).

The code for face-to-face behavioral counseling for obesity is a G0447 and is for a 15-minute counseling visit. The downside to this is that the current fee structure has this at $26.00. For nurse practitioners (since it is 85% of the physician fees schedule) the fee is ~$22 for 15-minute visit. This may not be a sustainable system for long-term financial health of a practice. This can be done in a group visit with up to 10 people for 30 minutes. The code for the group visit is G0473. The fee is $13/person so $130 ($110 for NPs) for the half hour if there are 10 people. Groups can be done with as few as 2, but still has to last 30 minutes. The same documentation has to occur for each patient. To complete the coding the Z code of BMI and counseling would be utilized.

General Documentation

Regardless of your billing decision the documentation around an obesity treatment plan must always include eating or dietary recommendations, activity recommendations, and what behavioral intervention you utilized. The documentation could include goal setting as this is behavioral counseling. If I am going to bill a medical visit it doesn't mean that I don't also document for their diabetes and hypertension. You will see in the example for timing that I do indeed document the complications and comorbidities.

Documentation and Billing Examples

TIMING (Example of the Assessment/Plan and Billing for the Visit)

Nancy is an established patient. She has returned at your request for a visit to discuss obesity.

Example of charting for the assessment and plan

Assessment:

1. Obesity E66.8 A/E BMI of 38.39 and waist circumference 51" Stage 2 based on BMI and obesity related complications.
2. E11.65 Diabetes A/E by HgbA1c 6.8—treating with management of obesity, metformin and SGLT2.
3. I10.0 Hypertension, controlled A/E by BP today of 128/86—treating with management of obesity and losartan.
4. F33.0 Depression—in remission A/E by PHQ9 of 4, continuing the antidepressant vortioxetine.
5. E78.1 Hypertriglyceridemia (new onset) —A/E by triglyceride of 230. Treating with management of obesity—will monitor with repeat level in 6 months.

Plan:

Patient here today for obesity appointment, seen for 30 minutes with 20 minutes for counseling.

Education completed on the disease of obesity.

Reviewed patient food tracking and types of food eating. Patient has set a SMART goal of reducing fast food by 50% —number of trips would then be less than 6 a week. She will add lunch items to her Sunday shopping list and each evening will pack her lunch when she packs her children's school lunches.

Sent requests for medical records to previous provider to get previous labs.

Patient to be seen again in 2 weeks.

Billing

- 99214
- E66.8 Obesity
- E11.65 Diabetes
- I10.0 Hypertension
- F33.0 Depression
- E78.1 Hypertriglyceridemia
- Z71.3

(If your system allows for more diagnosis, you could use more Z codes.)

Preventive Counseling Coding and Documentation

Let's take Nancy and make a change to code for preventive counseling

Assessment: (no changes here)

1. Obesity E66.8 A/E BMI of 38.395 and waist circumference 51" Stage 2 based on BMI and obesity related complications.
2. E11.65 Diabetes A/E by HgbA1c 6.8—treating with management of obesity and metformin and SGLT2.
3. I10.0 Hypertension, controlled A/E by BP today of 128/86—treating with management of obesity and medications (ACE-I).
4. F33.0 Depression—in remission A/E by PHQ9 of 4, continuing the antidepressant vortioxetine.
5. E78.1 Hypertriglyceridemia (new onset)—A/E by triglyceride of 230. Treating with management of obesity—will monitor with repeat level in 6 months.

Plan:

Patient is here today for obesity appointment, 20 minutes of counseling/education.

Education completed on the disease of obesity.

Reviewed patient's food tracking and types of food eating. Patient has SMART goal of reducing fast food by 50% number of trips would then be less than 6 a week. She will add lunch items to her Sunday shopping list and each evening will pack her lunch when she packs her children's school lunches.

Sent requests for medical records to previous provider to get previous labs.

Patient to be seen again in two weeks.

Billing:

- 99213 (being very sure that the history and physical meet this requirement—obviously with the 4 ORC there is medical complexity for this patient, but I am unlikely to meet the physical examination requirement for a 99214, thus the reason for the 99213)

- E66.8 Obesity
- E11.65 Diabetes
- I10.0 Hypertension
- F33.0 Depression
- E78.1 Hypertriglyceridemia
- Modifier 25 (if insurance has counseling available)
- 99401 (has 15 minutes of counseling—have 20 minutes documented but it goes in 15-minute blocks)
  - Z68.38
  - Z71.3

Preventive (Example of Assessment/Plan and Billing for the Visit)

Joe arrives as a new patient. He is 35 years old and wants to talk about his weight as he was told at his work that he should talk to his primary care about his weight. His measured height is 5′ 10″ and weight is 230. BMI is 33.0 kg/m^2 and his waist circumference is 43″. [Note: The history and physical will need to be comprehensive.]

Assessment:

BMI 33.0 kg/m^2 (*Do not code obesity* if doing preventive billing)

Plan: Reviewed patient's 3-day diet recall. Counseling completed about an eating plan. Patient has set first goal to decrease fast food eating for the next 2 weeks to only Monday and Friday. Will pack his lunch the other days during work week. Next visit for obesity treatment with counseling is in 2 weeks.

Billing:

- 99385 E&M code
- Z68.3 BMI
- Z13.89 Screening for obesity
- Z72.4 (Inappropriate diet and eating
- Z71.3 Dietary surveillance and counseling

Follow-Up Visit for Joe

Documentation in the HPI will include how Joe did with his goal. Today's weight is 227 so his BMI is 32.57.

Plan: Reviewed patient's 2-week food log. Counseling completed about decreasing ultraprocessed (UP) food, and patient has 4–6 servings of UP food daily. Assessed current activity and PARQ is negative. Patient met his first goal and will continue that as well starting to track his steps daily. Discussed the advantages of activity for general health. Patient has set his next two-week goal to decrease UP food to a maximum of 3 UP items a day. Provided handout to patient on how to identify UP food. Next visit for obesity treatment with counseling is in 2 weeks.

Assessment: Z68.32

Billing

- 99395 Preventative care follow-up
- Z68.32 BMI 32
- Z72.4 Inappropriate eating
- Z71.3 Counseling dietary
- Z71.89 Counseling exercise

[Authors note: after saying repeatedly that obesity is a chronic disease, this billing actually denies this by using prevention codes versus diagnosis. But it does provide the patient with no co-pay and additional income to the practice.]

MEDICARE IBT Documentation and Coding (Example of FU IBT)

Margaret is a 67-year-old with fee for service Medicare coverage. (She does have obesity, T2DM, HTN, and osteoarthritis, *but* for IBT those will NOT be addressed at today's visit).

Chief Complaint: Here for IBT based on initial BMI of 33.

Subjective: Patient states she tracked food for past week and has been walking for 5 minutes each day. She was able to increase vegetable servings to two times a day without any problems.

Objective: VS BP 132/84 HR 88 RR 16 pOx 95% Height 5′4″ wt 190 BMI today 32.61. Patient is alert and oriented, speaking in full sentences, respirations unlabored, skin normal color.

Assessment: BMI 33 (I keep this until the 6-month reevaluation)

Plan: 15 minutes face-to-face spent with patient for IBT. Assessed patient's food tracking and activity for the past week; found patient increasing intake of processed foods on Wednesday and Sunday with new job at church. Advised patient on healthier choices. Patient agreed to try new options at church social events. Assisted patient in creating new SMART Goal: increase walks to 10 minutes 3 days a week (Tuesday, Thursday, and Saturday) and continue at 5 minutes the other days. Arranged next IBT appointment in 1 week. 15 minutes spent with patient.

[Notice the five words for Medicare IBT are in the note: Assess, advise, agree, assist, arrange.]

Superbill

- G0447
- Z68.33
- Z13.89
- Z71.3

These examples are taken from patients in my clinical practice. As you can see you can get paid to treat the disease of obesity. So let that urban myth rest with the others.

Practice Pearls

- Insurances do pay for the treatment of obesity, not all yet but the majority.
- Coding doesn't have to be complicated and using known E&M coding is perfectly fine.
- Work with your billers and coders to determine if preventative codes are available.

References

1. Optum Coding. Evaluation and management coding advisor 2019. 2019. https://cdn.optumcoding.com/upload/pdf/EMCA19/EMCA_EMCA19%202019%20Sample%20Pages.pdf.
2. Healthcare.gov. Preventive care benefits for adults. https://www.healthcare.gov/preventive-care-adults/.
3. Contravehcp.com. Quick reference for common obesity-related ICD-10 codes. 2017. https://contravehcp.com/wp-content/uploads/2017/06/ICD_10_Reference_Guide.pdf.
4. Primary Care Obesity Management Certificate Program. ICD-10 codes for obesity management. n.d. https://www.aapa.org/wpcontent/uploads/2018/09/FINAL_Obesity_ICD10_Codes.pdf.
5. Department of Health and Human Services Centers for Medicare and Medicaid Services. Intensive behavioral therapy for obesity. 2012. https://www.cms.gov/Outreach-and-Education/Medicare-Learning-Network-MLN/MLNMattersArticles/downloads/MM7641.pdf.

Chapter 14
Putting It All Together in the Treatment of Obesity in Primary Care

BUT THOSE WERE THE COLDA-WOUL DA-SHOULDA'S ALL RAN AWAY FROM ONE LITTLE DID.

SHEF SILVERSTEIN

Key Reason

Integrating the components of obesity treatment into practice can seem overwhelming at first. But it really isn't. This chapter will look at a pattern of visits. Keep in mind that any of the education in visit 2 and on could be done by someone besides the provider in the practice.

Introduction

This chapter provides an overview of integrating all the learning from the previous chapters into practice. The preparation needed to ready a practice for treating patients with obesity is reviewed. A visit by visit recommendation for how to integrate the components of treatment into the primary care practice is provided.

A. Golden, *Treating Obesity in Primary Care*,
https://doi.org/10.1007/978-3-030-48683-9_14

Looking at obesity like we do any chronic disease makes it easy to identify the process. We can't treat it if we don't diagnose it (Step 1). We also need to determine the severity of the disease (Step 2) which includes any existing complication or comorbidities. Step 3 is to individualize the treatment to the patient based on history, physical assessment, and stage of the disease. This will include, at the least, treatment with the three components of selecting an eating plan, increasing physical activity, and behavioral intervention. It may also include pharmacology, referral for surgery, or consultation with an obesity specialist.

Preparation

Preparation means doing the scan of your practice. Are there any existing barriers—scale not in a private weighing area, appropriate reading material in the waiting room, chairs that accommodate a patient.

PRACTICE NOTE: Go back to the bias chapter and look at what needs checked in your practice and then go about getting it fixed.

Now that you have scanned your environment lets be sure *everyone* in the practice understands obesity as a disease not a lack of willpower or discipline. Each individual that documents in the patient's chart will need to have the permission to identify patients that need your help and notify you through a system approach. This is from the MA to all the other clinicians in your practice. This entails each person understanding that every patient with a BMI $\geq$ 25 kg/m^2 be evaluated for ORCs and get a waist circumference done at a visit that is not an urgent care type of visit. You know the patient, the one that comes in with a fever, nausea, and abdominal pain (or urinary frequency, or sore throat), this isn't the time to identify a chronic disease. But if the patient is there for a well visit OR a follow-up for med refills, both would be good times to assure the identification of patients at risk for obesity. The MA could flag the chart for you and other providers could do a referral.

PRACTICE NOTE: Don't forget the education that likely needs done on how to measure a waist circumference for visceral adiposity so that it is accurate.

In practice, here is what these recommendations would look like.

Visit Zero

- Patient is identified as being at risk for obesity based on BMI ≥25 kg/m^2/Asian ≥23 kg/m^2 (assure height was measure in stocking feet—not stated).
- Measure waist circumference for patients with BMI 25–35 kg/m^2.
  - High-risk for cardiometabolic abnormalities: >88 cm/35 inches in women and >102 cm/40 inches in men (Asian females, waist circumference >80 cm (31.5 inches) and in Asian males a value >90 cm (35.4 inches).
- Provider providing obesity care is notified of potential and evaluates for documented obesity-related complications.
- Provider asks* the patient for permission to talk about weight and obesity.
- Make a follow-up visit to do a full obesity evaluation
  - Send obesity intake paperwork with the patient (or sent to them if they prefer). This includes the AACE intake and obesity-related complication (ORC) form. Of course, if the patient is already part of your practice you won't need insurance information or past medical history – but it is great to use this even if some is repetitive to help patients get a view of obesity as a chronic disease before they come in to see you.

*Ask

Ask the patients permission to talk about their weight. As I mentioned you could have handouts in the practice and every room to explain the treatment options and the disease of obesity. Once the patient has agreed to discuss the disease use your 30 second to 2 minute explanation of the disease and an overview of the components of treatment. Then make a follow-up appointment for a full obesity evaluation and start of a treatment plan. I recommend this follow-up visit be only to discuss obesity and schedule for 40 minutes if at all possible.

Visit One for Obesity

Assess

Patient history

- History of weight gain and loss overtime (see weight history Fig. 14.1)
- Details of previous weight loss attempts including previous anti-obesity medications or over the counter substances
- Current eating habits—ask about any food sensitivities or allergies
- Current physical activity

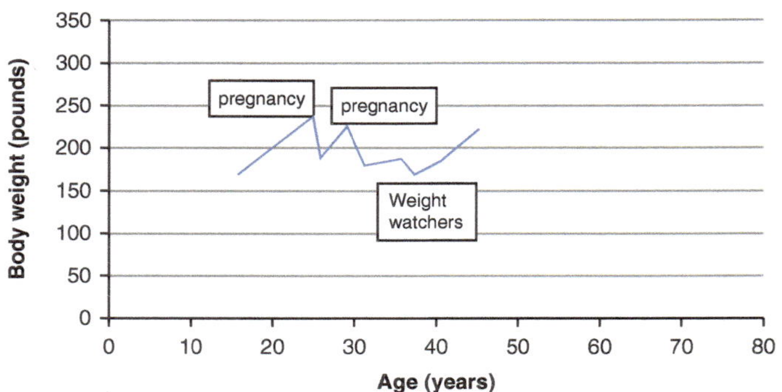

FIGURE 14.1 Weight body graph

- Current medications:
  - specifically, to identify any obesogenic medications that may need changed
  - medications that would interact with anti-obesity medications
- Current medical problems—evaluating for obesity-related complications or comorbidities (for staging of disease as well as assistance with medication selection) that treating obesity could impact
  - Each note going forward mentions them
- Alcohol and illicit drug use—alcohol use can impact medication choices
- Smoking history—recent cessation can add to weight gain
- PMH
  - Hx of stroke, cardiovascular disease, arteriosclerosis, valvular heart disease, uncontrolled hypertension, glaucoma, hyperthyroidism, seizures, renal disease, pulmonary hypertension, and/or pancreatitis. Each of these can assist in choosing medication management if that becomes part of the treatment plan (which it does in 80–90% of my patients).

Family history
- Overweight or obesity
- Family history of thyroid cancer (I just ask about any thyroid cancer and if the answer is yes, then I have patients find out the type—the most common thyroid cancer is papillary. Rarely do patients know the type so I ask them to investigate this since medullary thyroid cancer would be a contraindication to a GLP-1 agonist).

PRACTICE NOTE: Many of my patients have done the weight loss clinics that use the non-evidence-based practice of vitamin injections, Human Chorionic Gonadotropin and 500 calorie diets. Generally, the patient who has done a weight loss clinic also has experience with higher dose of phentermine 37.5 mg.

TABLE 14.1 Physical examination findings and indications

Physical exam specific to obesity	Finding	Indicates possibility of
Skin	Rashes in skin folds Hirsutism in women Acanthosis nigricans	Possible fungal infections Excess testosterone or possible Polycystic Ovarian Syndrome Insulin resistance
Cardiovascular	Irregular heart rate PMI shifted Decreased diaphragmatic excursion	Possible arrhythmias like atrial fibrillation Cardiomegaly Respiratory insufficiency
Respiratory	Decreased diaphragmatic excursion	Respiratory insufficiency
Abdomen	Enlarged liver measurement Striae	Nonalcoholic fatty liver disease possibility Excess cortisol
Extremities	Peripheral edema or varicosities Joint deformities	Congestive Heart Failure, Peripheral Vascular Disease Pressure alterations, arthritis
General	Lipodystrophic fat distribution	Insulin resistant

Physical Examination (Table 14.1)

Vital Signs

Screening Tools

- PHQ9—screen for depression since many AOMs can have an impact and it is a comorbidity—presence of either worsens the other.
- BED-7—evaluations for binge eating, 30% of patients with obesity have BED as well and will require treatment for this psychiatric disorder with obesity treatment. At this

time assess for eating disorders screening for purging behaviors.

- STOP BANG—screening for sleep apnea, a comorbidity with obesity, they each worsen the other, and PARQ.

Diagnostics (to Assess for ORCs or Complications)

Complete blood count, Comprehensive metabolic panel, Thyroid stimulating hormone with FT4 and FT3, Vitamin D, lipid panel, fasting insulin (or c-peptide) and fasting glucose. Fasting insulin or c-peptide with the fasting glucose will be placed into the HOMA-IR2 calculator to evaluate for insulin resistance *if* the patient does not have established prediabetes or diabetes.

PRACTICE NOTE: Be sure to ask the patient what they think their obstacle is to maintain optimal health. This brings them into the conversation *and* most often you hear—not enough willpower, not enough time to work out. This is where you can start to change their paradigm on what it takes to treat the disease. Yes, there are behavioral components, but it is a medical diagnosis and there are options to support their behavior changes.

Diagnose and Stage

- Using either AACE or EOSS stage the disease

Plan

- Make any referrals that need to be made.
  - Examples include clearance for activity, sleep study, or physical therapy.
- Additional assessment for next visit—ask the patient to track their intake and current physical activity.
- Make the next several follow-up appointments within 2–3 weeks of each other.

PRACTICE NOTE: One thing to think about as you're setting all of this up is to be sure that you have openings in your schedule for these follow-up visits.

Visit Two—Initiating Obesity Treatment Plan

- History
  - Review food tracking
  - Review physical activity tracking
- Physical Examination
  - VS
  - Minimal physical is needed
- Assessment and diagnosis
  - Identify obesity code and any ORCs
- Plan
  - Set short-term and long-term goals of treatment
  - Select an eating plan or begin making modifications of eating (ex: decreasing fast food intake)—make a SMART goal
  - Monitor hunger
  - Discuss possibility of medication, possible need to change an obesogenic medication, and/or surgery referrals
  - Educational handout related to obesity and treatment

PRACTICE NOTE: Discuss the patients *why* for treatment. This helps guide the evaluation moving forward. Our goal is 5–10% weight loss to impact obesity-related complications, and the patients goal may be to allow them to be more active with their children.

Visit Three

- History
  - Review food tracking and SMART goal from previous visit—any roadblocks to meeting the goal
  - Review any needed information related to ORCs (e.g., patient has diabetes and you review blood sugar logs)

- Physical Examination
  - VS
  - Minimal physical is needed
- Assessment and diagnosis
  - Identify obesity code and any ORCs
- Plan
  - Revisit eating decisions—modifications with smart goals versus meal plan
  - Create new SMART goal around eating for next 2 weeks
  - Determine patients desire to go to medications if patient is tracking food well then this will be addressed at this visit or next visit
  - Evaluate if any plan is needed for any ORCs you assessed
  - ILI—select an education handout for today—5-minute review of the handout

Visit Four

- History
  - Review food tracking and SMART goal from previous visit—any roadblocks to meeting the goal, if so ask patient what prevented them from meeting their goal
  - Review any needed information related to ORCs (e.g., depression—new PHQ9 to assure still in remission)
- Physical Examination
  - VS
  - Minimal physical is needed
- Assessment and diagnosis
  - Identify obesity code and any ORCs
- Plan
  - Revisit eating decisions—modifications with smart goals versus meal plan—problem solve for any road-

blocks and create new SMART goal around eating for next 2 week
- Two options
  - Start Activity discussion (if doing this then set a SMART goal) or
  - Select medication and order (or start prior authorization)
- Evaluate if any plan is needed for any ORCs you assessed
- ILI – select an education handout for today—5-minute review of the handout

Visit Five

- History
  - Review food tracking and SMART goal from previous visit—any roadblocks to meeting the goal, if so ask patient what prevented them from meeting their goal
  - Check for SE of medication—evaluate hunger on the beginning dose, if not improved, then increase dose if medication selected has dose changes
  - Review any needed information related to ORCs (e.g., depression—new PHQ9 to assure still in remission)
- Physical Examination
  - VS
  - Minimal physical is needed
- Assessment and diagnosis
  - Identify obesity code and any ORCs
- Plan
  - Revisit eating decisions—modifications with smart goals versus meal plan—problem solve for any roadblocks and create new SMART goal around eating for next 2 week

- Two options—if started medication, then go to activity discussion
    - Start Activity discussion (if doing this then set a SMART goal) or
    - Select medication and order (or start prior authorization)
- Evaluate if any plan is needed for any ORCs you assessed
- ILI—select an education handout for today—5-minute review of the handout

Visit Six On Continues in the Same Way

- Evaluate patients' SMART goals, helping to determine behavior changes that may be needed
- Evaluate patient is losing weight—if on medication, as you approach week 12 at the maximum dose, assure the 4–5% weight loss, if not will need to change medication
- Evaluate impact of obesity treatment on patients ORCs being prepared to change any ORC medication management

Practice Profiles

There are many ways to integrate obesity into primary care practice. Following are just a few but you can likely see many other options for your practice.

Primary Care Integration

Using your chronic care model obesity treatment would be integrated into every non-sickness visit. Early in treatment there will need to be frequent visits based on what we have learned from the research. These visits can be with the prescriber (NP, PA, physician) or perhaps others in your practice (e.g., social worker, dietician, nurses, or exercise expert). One thing to keep in mind, each of these individuals must understand obesity as a disease. Think of treating a patient with a new diagnosis of diabetes, you would rarely do all this alone but would use others in your practice or community.

Dedicated Day(s) for Obesity

Several primary care practices I have worked with have identified one clinician/prescriber to see all newly diagnosed patients with obesity on a specific day to allow the prescriber to become very proficient. Patients then become comfortable with walking into the practice.

Regardless of the system that you select, the goal for the practice should be congruent with every other chronic disease treatment. Improve patient health and quality of life by preventing or treating obesity-related complications.

Practice Pearls

- During the history and physical you are also looking for secondary causes of obesity; Cushings, genetic syndromes, obesogenic medications, recent smoking cessation, and don't forget to test for pregnancy as it is a cause of weight gain.
- Recognize other providers that can support the obesity treatment team.
- This is a journey in a chronic, relapsing, *and* treatable disease, so partner with your patient to provide long-term care.

Chapter 15
Example in Clinic

LIFE ISN'T ABOUT FINDING YOURSELF. LIFE IS ABOUT CREATING YOURSELF.

GEORGE BERNARD SHAW

Key Reason
Treating obesity in primary care means treating this disease with many others. This chapter will follow several patients in primary care with the evidence-based treatment that has been reviewed in this book.

Introduction

This chapter utilizes two patients and follows their care through the continuum of treatment in a practice. These cases demonstrate the intricacies of integrating obesity with other chronic care issues for patients and include the documentation and billing utilized from real practice cases.

A. Golden, *Treating Obesity in Primary Care*,
https://doi.org/10.1007/978-3-030-48683-9_15

Ashley

Ashley is a 42-year-old who works part-time as a banker. She was into the practice for a checkup and refill on her citalopram.

- Medical Assistant (MA) measures patient 5′3″ and weight 192# BMI 34 kg/m^2
  - MA takes patient into the room and explains that there is a new measurement for the practice—waist measurement 44″.
  - MA flags the chart for the Nurse Practitioner that patient meets the parameters for obesity discussion.
- Patient is evaluated for depression—PHQ9 score 4, and patient reports no side effects from citalopram, refill provided for antidepressant.
- NP asks permission to speak to patient about her weight. "Ashley, I notice that your weight is up a bit from your last appointment. I would like to talk with you about treatment options if you would be okay with that?" The patient readily says yes and a follow-up appointment is made and patient is provided with paperwork to complete for her next appointment.

Visit One for Obesity

Patient History

- Has tried multiple times to lose weight, feels she has always been heavy. She tried phentermine in the past for weight loss but did not tolerate the side effects; she did not like feeling jittery. She also tried orlistat and several OTC herbs. She did not tolerate the side effects of orlistat and stopped it after 2 weeks. She has not reached her weight loss goal in any attempt. And when she has lost weight, she gains it back (Fig. 15.1). She tells you she's tried to lose

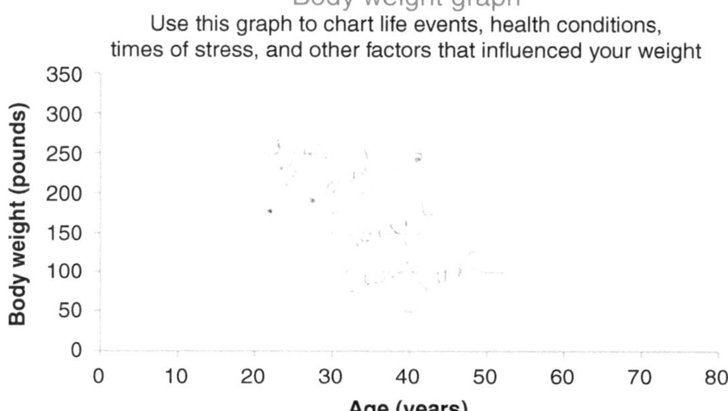

FIGURE 15.1 Body weight graph

weight many, many times at least six or seven for prolonged periods. She does lose 20–30 pounds with attempts but gains it back again. She's tired of it and she's frustrated.

- Used this as a teaching time to talk about obesity as a disease and metabolic adaptation.
- Current eating habits—ask about any food sensitivities or allergies—She feels like she's always thinking about food especially sweets and snacks. She finds it hard to curb her cravings instead of eating only a few chips. She will eat ½ of a regular size bag.
- Current physical activity—nothing specific—"walk a lot at work"
- Current medications: ibuprofen, citalopram
- Pregnancy prevention program: IUD
- Current medical problems
  - Sleep apnea, reports intermittent use of her CPAP
  - Gastroesophageal reflux disease that is treated with protonix

- Osteoarthritis of both knees that she takes ibuprofen prn
- Depression which she says is treated successfully with citalopram

Social History

- She lives with her husband and two daughters
- She drinks socially maybe one glass of wine per week and she denies any illicit drug use
- No history of use of tobacco

PMH: Denies history of stroke, cardiovascular disease, arteriosclerosis, valvular heart disease, uncontrolled hypertension, glaucoma, hyperthyroidism, seizures, renal disease, pulmonary hypertension, or pancreatitis.

Family History: Both parents alive. Father is 72—HTN and MI at age of 62; mother is 70 with Type 2 Diabetes. Brother is alive with hypothyroidism. Reports no family history of thyroid cancer.

ROS General: generally able to accomplish all activities of daily living, no change in strength or exercise tolerance. Head: No headaches, no vertigo. Eyes: Normal vision, no diplopia. Chest: No dyspnea. Heart: No chest pains, no palpitations, no syncope, no orthopnea. Abdomen: no dysphagia, no abdominal pains, no bowel habit changes, no emesis. Neurologic: No weakness, no tremor, no seizures, no changes in mentation. Psychiatric: No depressive symptoms, no changes in sleep habits, no changes in thought content. Sleep–wakes feeling rested when using CPAP. Pain—occasional knee pain.

Physical Exam

VS: BP 122/80 HR 78 RR 16 pOx 98% 5′3″ 192# BMI 34 kg/m^2

Objective General: patient in NAD, cooperative with examiner, well groomed, alert and oriented × 4.

Eyes: PERRL, Eyes: conjunctivae clear, no discharge. Ears: Canals clear bilaterally, TM's normal bilaterally. Nose: Moist, pink mucosa without lesions or mass. Throat: no exudates, no erythema.

Neck: Supple, no masses, no thyromegaly, no bruits, no lymphadenopathy.

Chest: BSCTA = bil, no rales, no rhonchi, no wheezes, speaking in full sentences, respirations non labored.

Heart/CV: RR, no rubs, no gallops; Radial and pedal pulses 2+ = bil.

Abdomen: bowel sounds normal, percussion tones nl, SNT without rebound, no masses, no hepatomegaly or splenomegaly.

Neuro: A&O × 4, CN II-XII grossly intact, stable gait, Romberg negative, DTR's 2+ and = bilaterally, recent and distant memory grossly intact.

Extremities: Warm, well perfused, no edema, grips and pushes 2+ = bilaterally.

Screenings completed: BED- 7 SCORE: negative. STOPBANG: Not done as patient has diagnosis of Sleep Apnea PHQ9 Score of 4 PARQ negative.

Recent labs show her CMP, CBC, TSH, FT4, and FT3 are within normal range. Total cholesterol is 245, LDL is 134, triglycerides 273, HDL 38, and her hemoglobin A-1 C is 5.8.

Chart Note

Diagnose and Stage

According to AACE, Ashley has obesity. Her BMI is 34 kg/m^2 with a waist circumference of 44″, which represents excess visceral adiposity, and she has several obesity-related complications (prediabetes, GERD, hyperlipidemia, osteoarthritis) and comorbidities (depression and OSA). These place her at diagnostic stage 2.

- Ashley Jones 42 years.
- Diagnosis of obesity Stage 2 E66.8 based on BMI of 34 and ORCs.
- E78.2 Mixed Hyperlipidemia as evidenced by Total cholesterol is 245, LDL is 134, triglycerides 273, HDL 38. Her ASCVD is 1.9%. Will treat the hyperlipidemia with treatment of obesity with risk so low, no statin at this time.
- R73.03 Prediabetes—as evidenced by HgBA1C of 5.8. Will treat with weight loss and reevaluate at 5% weight loss—starting metformin 500 mg q day for 2 weeks will review dosing at next visit.
- K21.9 GERD—as evidenced by reflux sx controlled currently with protonix. Obesity treatment should improve this—after 10% weight loss will do a trial of removing medication for GERD.
- M17.9 OA, knees—treats with prn ibuprofen—recommend change to Tylenol due to GERD and will monitor with 5% weight loss for improvement.
- Complications
  - F32.2 Major Depression Disorder—as evidenced by previous PHQ9 of 11 and now controlled at 4 and treatment with citalopram. Will monitor this closely at each visit.
  - G47.33 sleep apnea—patient reports using CPAP 3–4 nights/week, further treatment with obesity treatment and weight loss. Patient agrees to use nightly after understanding of benefits for sleep for obesity. Will order a new sleep test after patient has a 10% weight loss.
- Met with patient for 40 minutes, completed intake history and physical examination, and did education on the disease of obesity.
- No referrals needed based on screening.
- Discussed currently recommended obesity management strategies.

- Introduction to the practice with the My Fitness Pal will send connection information and the importance of tracking.
- Education on obesity as a disease.
- Plan for next visit:
  - Track on My Fitness Pal.
  - Patient will be monitoring intake very closely so will review this at the next visit.
  - Decision on food plan choice will be made—patient was given handout on eating plan options.
  - Tracking steps for next 2 weeks.
  - Next visit in 2 weeks.

[Practice note: In summary, Ashley's evaluation demonstrates a diagnosis of obesity, mild depression, GERD, sleep apnea, osteoarthritis, and new diagnosis of hyperlipidemia and prediabetes. She is a long history of weight loss and regain and complains of cravings for sweet and salty snacks. She has tried orlistat and phentermine 37.5 mg with SE that were not tolerable in the past. She has repeated attempts at weight loss.]

This visit was coded as follows:

- E&M 99215—patient with provider for 40 minutes with significant history and physical and medical complexity
  - ICD10 E66.8
  - G47.33 Sleep apnea
  - K21.9 GERD
  - F32.2 Major Depression Disorder
  - R73.03 Prediabetes
  - E78.2 Mixed Hyperlipidemia
  - M17.9 OA, knees

Visit 2–22

	Visit Two	Visit Three
HX	Review food tracking: She is averaging 1600 calories a day, finds that about 400 calories are after dinner, and she doesn't feel full at any time during the day Review physical activity tracking—Her average steps are 5500/day Denies any change in depression symptoms Patient denies any side effects with Metformin Patient has noticed no change in GERD symptoms Knee pain remains stable, pain is mostly on days when she is sitting more than walking Reports has been using CPAP every night, is feeling somewhat more rested	Review food tracking: She is averaging 1500 calories a day, CHO 250 g/day, Protein 48 g/day Notices a significant decrease of hunger through the day but evenings are still difficult. Patient reports eating fast food three times in the past 2 weeks and continuing to decrease processed foods Review physical activity tracking—Reports average steps are 6500/day Taking Contrave one tablet twice a day Metformin is at one tablet twice a day Denies any side effects of Contrave or metformin Continues to use CPAP every night
ROS	*General*: Patient denies change in exercise tolerance. Denies insomnia *Lungs*: Patient denies SOB w usual activity and Shortness of breath at rest *Heart*: Patient denies Palpitations, Irregular heart beat and Chest pains. *GI*: Patient denies Changes in way food taste or loss of taste, Dry mouth, Abdominal pain, Nausea, Vomiting, Diarrhea, and Constipation *Neurologic*: Patient denies Headache, Numbness in extremities and Dizziness. *Psychiatric*: Patient denies Suicidal thoughts and Depression *Endocrine*: Patient denies Excessive thirst or hunger	*General*: Patient denies change in exercise tolerance. Denies insomnia *Lungs*: Patient denies SOB w usual activity and Shortness of breath at rest *Heart*: Patient denies Palpitations, Irregular heartbeat, and Chest pains *Abdomen*: Patient denies Changes in way food taste or loss of taste, Dry mouth, Abdominal pain, Nausea, Vomiting, Diarrhea, and Constipation *Neurologic*: Patient denies Headache, Numbness in extremities, and Dizziness *Psychiatric*: Patient denies Suicidal thoughts and Depression *Endocrine*: Patient denies Excessive thirst or hunger

PE	VS: BP 118/74 HR 82 RR 16 pOx 98% 5′3″ 188# BMI 33.3 kg/m^2. Patient is alert and oriented × 4, recent and remote memory intact. Breathing is non-labored, patient speaking in full sentences. Radial pulse has RRR. Skin is normal color, cap refill is <2 seconds. Gait is normal. PHQ9 4	VS: BP 120/76 HR 80 RR 16 pOx 98% 5′3″ 186# BMI 32.94 kg/m2. Patient is alert and oriented × 4, recent and remote memory intact. Breathing is non-labored, patient speaking in full sentences. Radial pulse has RRR. Skin is normal color, cap refill is <2 seconds. Gait is normal. PHQ9 4
DX	Diagnosis of obesity Stage 2 E66.8 based on BMI of 33.3 original BMI 34 and ORCs R73.03 Prediabetes—as evidenced by HgBA1C of 5.8. Will treat with weight loss and reevaluate at 5% weight loss—metformin to be increased to twice a day 500 mg for 2 weeks will review dosing at next visit K21.9 GERD—as evidenced by reflux sx controlled currently with protonix. Obesity treatment should improve this—after 10% weight loss will do a trial of removing medication for GERD M17.9 OA, knees—treats with prn ibuprofen – recommend change to Tylenol due to GERD and will monitor with 5% weight loss for improvement F32.2 Major Depression Disorder—as evidenced by previous PHQ9 of 11 and now controlled at 4 and treatment with citalopram. Will monitor this closely at each visit G47.33 sleep apnea—patient reports using CPAP every night, further treatment with obesity treatment and weight loss. Patient agrees to use nightly after understanding of benefits for sleep for obesity. Will order a new sleep test after patient has a 10% weight loss	Diagnosis of obesity Stage 2 E66.8 based on BMI of 32.94 original BMI 34 and ORCs R73.03 Prediabetes—as evidenced by HgBA1C of 5.8. Will treat with weight loss and reevaluate at 5% weight loss—metformin to be increased to twice a day 500 mg for 2 weeks will review dosing at next visit K21.9 GERD—as evidenced by reflux sx controlled currently with protonix. Obesity treatment should improve this—after 10% weight loss will do a trial of removing medication for GERD M17.9 OA, knees—treats with prn ibuprofen—recommend change to Tylenol due to GERD and will monitor with 5% weight loss for improvement F32.2 Major Depression Disorder—as evidenced by previous PHQ9 of 11 and now controlled at 4 and treatment with citalopram. Will monitor this closely at each visit G47.33 sleep apnea—patient reports using CPAP every night, further treatment with obesity treatment and weight loss. Patient agrees to use nightly after understanding of benefits for sleep for obesity. Will order a new sleep test after patient has a 10% weight loss

(continued)

	Visit Two	Visit Three
Plan	Met with patient for 25 minutes, 20 minutes in counseling and education Ashley says her goal is to be healthier. [with motivational interviewing this is further detailed] She wants wake feeling rested and be able to run a 5 K with her family and wear a size 12 pants. Goals from a health perspective could include eliminating or minimizing obesity-related complications and comorbidities which should be seen at about 5–10% weight loss. Ashley agrees with this plan Discussed eating plans and patient states would like to reduce processed foods. SMART GOAL: will limit fast food to two times a week and pack her lunch the evening before to take to work Medication management decision: discussed medication options, patient does not have any contraindication for any medication, has no insurance coverage for medications leaving out liraglutide due to cost. Due to cravings will start Contrave and order placed with mail order pharmacy. Patient to start one tablet per day, if no side effects can move to one tablet bid in 1 week. Pregnancy prevention informed consent signed. Patient verbalized understanding of need to continue pregnancy prevention with IUD. Patient provided with medication handout, reviewed with no questions Follow-up plan for this visit: Continue to Track intake on My Fitness Pal Track hunger and satiety (provided with handout) with start of anti-obesity medication Increase metformin to 500 mg bid Contrave 8 mg/90 mg one tablet each morning, if no side effects may increase to one tablet bid until next visit Follow-up appointment in 2 weeks Email or call with any concerns Education at this appointment mindfulness around eating and medication	Met with patient for 25 minutes, 20 minutes in counseling and education Last SMART goal was met—ate out less than 4 times at fast food over 2 weeks and packed lunch Discussed continued eating changes. Patient will continue to decrease processed foods. Reviewed the value of protein. Patient decided to have SMART goal for the next 2 weeks: Increase protein to 80 g/day and 30 grams for breakfast using a pea protein shake daily Activity plan: Discussed the need to continue to increase activity since by maintenance will need to be at 250–300 minutes per week. SMART goal: increase steps to 7000 on Monday, Wednesday and Friday Medication management: increase Contrave to two tablets in afternoon and hold with one tablet in the am. Pregnancy prevention remains in place Patient provided with handouts on protein grams in food and protein snacks Follow-up plan for this visit: Continue to track intake on My Fitness Pal Increase Contrave 8 mg/90 mg one tablet each morning and two in the afternoon. Monitor hunger and satiety SMART goal for the next 2 weeks: Increase protein to 80 g/day and 30 grams for breakfast using a pea protein shake daily. SMART goal: increase steps to 7000 on Monday, Wednesday and Friday Follow-up appointment in 2 weeks Email or call with any concerns Education at this appointment use of protein

Billing	99214 (time) ICD10 E66.8 Obesity G47.33 Sleep apnea K21.9 GERD F32.2 Major Depression Disorder R73.03 Prediabetes E78.2 Mixed Hyperlipidemia M17.9 OA, knees Z71.3 Dietary surveillance and counseling Z71.89 Exercise counseling	99214 (time) ICD10 E66.8 Obesity G47.33 Sleep apnea F32.2 Major Depression Disorder Z71.3 Dietary surveillance and counseling Z71.89 Exercise counseling

	Visit Four	**Visit Five**	**Visit Six—22**
HX	Review food tracking: She is averaging 1300 calories a day, CHO 175 g/day, Protein 80 g/day—has no fast food for past 2 weeks. Breakfast 10 days out of 14 with 30 g of protein—not reaching this on Saturday and Sunday Notices a significant decrease of hunger through the day and no longer eating in the evening except on weekends Review physical activity tracking—Reports average steps are 7000/day. Taking Contrave one tablet in am and two in late afternoon Metformin is at one tablet twice a day Denies any side effects of Contrave or metformin Continues to use CPAP every night	Review food tracking: She is averaging 1300 calories a day, CHO 150 g/day, Protein 90 g/day— continues with no fast food. Breakfast 14 days out of 14 with 30 g of protein Notices a significant decrease of hunger and states feels in control of eating and choices now Review physical activity tracking—Reports average steps are 8000/5 days a week. Started with trainer for weight resistance Has not had to use any ibuprofen in the past 2 weeks as knees have not been hurting at all Taking Contrave one tablet in am and two in late afternoon Metformin is at one tablet twice a day Denies any side effects of Contrave or metformin Continues to use CPAP every night	Continue to review food tracking and any roadblocks with shared decision-making to get around them Monitor medication and side effects At 1 year walking is at 10,000–15,000 steps a day with 3 × week weight resistance training No longer uses ibuprofen or protonix Dose of Contrave and metformin remained stable with no side effects CPAP stopped by sleep specialist when patient reevaluated at 18% weight loss At 1 year trial off antidepressant

(continued)

	Visit Four	Visit Five	Visit Six – 22
ROS	*General*: Patient denies change in exercise tolerance. Denies insomnia *Lungs*: Patient denies SOB w usual activity and shortness of breath at rest *Heart*: Patient denies Palpitations, Irregular heartbeat, and Chest pains *Abdomen*: Patient denies Changes in way food taste or loss of taste, Dry mouth, Abdominal pain, Nausea, Vomiting, Diarrhea, and Constipation *Neurologic*: Patient denies Headache, Numbness in extremities, and Dizziness *Psychiatric*: Patient denies Suicidal thoughts and Depression *Endocrine*: Patient denies Excessive thirst or hunger	*General*: Patient denies change in exercise tolerance. Denies insomnia *Lungs*: Patient denies SOB w usual activity and shortness of breath at rest *Heart*: Patient denies Palpitations, Irregular heartbeat, and Chest pains *Abdomen*: Patient denies Changes in way food taste or loss of taste, Dry mouth, Abdominal pain, Nausea, Vomiting, Diarrhea, and Constipation *Neurologic*: Patient denies Headache, Numbness in extremities, and Dizziness *Psychiatric*: Patient denies Suicidal thoughts and Depression *Endocrine*: Patient denies Excessive thirst or hunger	*Continue ROS for each visit*

PE	VS: BP 120/76 HR 80 RR 16 pOx 98% 5′3″ 182# BMI 32.24 kg/m^2. Patient is alert and oriented × 4, recent and remote memory intact. Breathing is non-labored, patient speaking in full sentences. Radial pulse has RRR. Skin is normal color, cap refill is <2 seconds Gait is normal. PHQ9 4	VS: BP 116/72 HR 72 RR 16 pOx 98% 5′3″ 178# BMI 31.53 kg/m^2 Patient is alert and oriented × 4, recent and remote memory intact. Breathing is non-labored, patient speaking in full sentences. Radial pulse has RRR. Skin is normal color, cap refill is <2 seconds Gait is normal. PHQ9 2	Continues visits on regular basis every 2–3 weeks End of year one VS: BP 112/68 HR 72 RR 16 pOx 98% 5′3″ 153.6 # Waist circumference 35" BMI 31.53 kg/m^2. BMI 27.10 Patient is alert and oriented × 4, recent and remote memory intact. Breathing is non-labored, patient speaking in full sentences. Radial pulse has RRR. Skin is normal color, cap refill is <2 seconds. Gait is normal. PHQ9 2 Lipid panel tested at 1 year—all levels in normal range HgBA1C 5.2
DX	99214 (time) ICD10 E66.8 Obesity G47.33 Sleep apnea F32.2 Major Depression Disorder R73.03 Prediabetes E78.2 Mixed Hyperlipidemia M17.9 OA, knees Z71.3 Dietary surveillance and counseling Z71.89 Exercise counseling	99214 (time) ICD10 E66.8 Obesity G47.33 Sleep apnea K21.9 GERD F32.2 Major Depression Disorder R73.03 Prediabetes E78.2 Mixed Hyperlipidemia M17.9 OA, knees Z71.3 Dietary surveillance and counseling Z71.89 Exercise counseling	99214 (time) ICD10 E66.8 Obesity (at 1 year now stage 1 versus stage 2) F32.2 Major Depression Disorder Z71.3 Dietary surveillance and counseling Z71.89 Exercise counseling

(continued)

	Visit Four	Visit Five	Visit Six – 22
Plan	Met with patient for 25 minutes, 20 minutes in counseling and education Last SMART goal was met—ate out less than 4 times at fast food over 2 weeks and packed lunch Discussed continued eating changes Patient will continue to decrease processed foods Patient decided to have SMART goal for the next 2 weeks: 30 grams of protein for breakfast to continue On upcoming holiday will track food before eating it to keep carbohydrates under 200 and calories below 1800 for the day Activity plan: Discussed the need to continue to increase activity since by maintenance will need to be at 250–300 minutes per week. SMART goal: increase steps to 7500 on Monday, Wednesday, Friday, and Saturday Medication management: Has met the 5% requirement to continue medication and has decrease in hunger noticed as well as fewer cravings at night Pregnancy prevention remains in place Patient provided with handouts holiday eating and serving size	Met with patient for 25 minutes, 20 minutes in counseling and education Last SMART goal was met: 30 grams of protein for breakfast to continue. On upcoming holiday will track food before eating it to keep carbohydrates under 200 and calories below 1800 for the day SMART goal met increase steps to 7500 on Monday, Wednesday, Friday, and Saturday Discussed importance of long-term food tracking Patient decided to have SMART goal for the next 2 weeks: Remain with protein to 80 g/day and 30 g for breakfast using a pea protein shake daily Activity plan: SMART goal: increase steps to 8500 steps on Monday, Wednesday, Friday, and Sunday Medication management: increase Contrave to remain at one tablet in the am and two in the afternoon. Pregnancy prevention remains in place Reviewed patients "Why of treatment" she is planning to walk a 5 K—has registered for one in 2 weeks, is wearing a size 14, and very excited about this	Once at 173# will need to reassess sleep apnea with referral to sleep lab and a trial off protonix Throughout this time continue with education at each visit At one-year plan going forward: Stopped metformin, protonix, and ibuprofen Continue tracking food intake Continue and increase steps Continue anaerobic activity Continue Contrave See patient every 3 months, unless weight regain of 5 pounds then to come in sooner

Plan	Follow-up plan for this visit: Continue to Track intake on My Fitness Pal Continue Contrave 8 mg/90 mg one tablet each morning and two in the afternoon. Monitor hunger and satiety SMART goal for the next 2 weeks: 30 g of protein for breakfast to continue. On upcoming holiday will track food before eating it to keep carbohydrates under 200 and calories below 1800 for the day SMART goal: increase steps to 7500 on Monday, Wednesday, Friday, and Saturday Follow-up appointment in 2 weeks Email or call with any concerns Education at this appointment how to plan ahead for upcoming holiday and serving size	Patient provided with handouts Events and Challenges and discussed the items to be aware of that at this point can cause issues for stalling the forward progress Follow-up plan for this visit: Continue to Track intake on My Fitness Pal Increase Contrave 8 mg/90 mg one tablet each morning and two in the afternoon. Monitor hunger and satiety SMART goal for the next 2 weeks: Remain with protein to 80 g/day and 30 g for breakfast using a pea protein shake daily. SMART goal: increase steps to 8500 steps on Monday, Wednesday, Friday, and Sunday Follow-up appointment in 2 weeks Email or call with any concerns Education at this appointment use of Events and Challenges

Susan

Susan, a 28-year-old, is here today for follow-up on her new migraine treatment. BMI is of 33 kg/m^2. The MA does a waist and neck measurement after the patient is in the room. (After assuring the patient does not have a headache of course.) An alert is placed on the chart for the positive screen for obesity. You see the waist circumference of 40 inches and next circumference of 15 inches. You proceed with the headache evaluation noting she's only needed one rescue med in the past month since the neurologist started her on propranolol 40 mg daily. She does state that she's noticed a 5-pound weight gain in the past 2 months and is more tired at dinnertime. She's removed all caffeine based on the recommendation she was given previously for migraine prevention. You obtain the characteristics of her headache that required abortive medication. She did bring up her weight gain. I would say, "Susan, you mentioned the weight gain and our records indicate numbers of another chronic disease. It is called obesity. I would like to talk to you about your weight and what treatments are available and how this might help your headaches as well." Susan quickly agreed. Here is a sample elevator speech: "Obesity is a chronic disease. It isn't a personal failing or will power issue. It has endocrine, hormonal and pathology problems." Of course, depending on the patients' health literacy, you may need to use slightly different words. Makes a visit in 2 weeks for Visit One for Obesity.

Visit One for Obesity

Patient History

- Has tried multiple times to lose weight, feels she has always been heavy. She has never tried any medications or

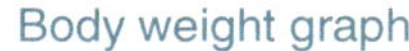

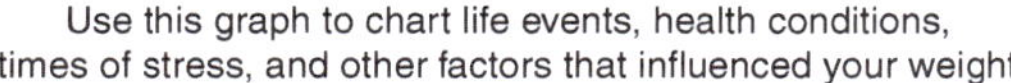

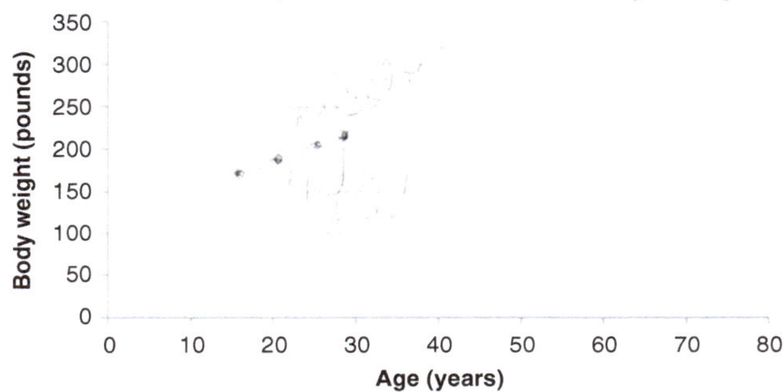

FIGURE 15.2 Body weight graph

over the counter things like herbs. She has always lost 15–20 pounds but then gains back 20–25 pounds (Fig. 15.2).

- Current eating habits—patient states she hates cooking and eating alone so frequently 10–15 times a week grabs fast food on her way home from work and at lunchtime. Has no food allergies or sensitivities.
- Current physical activity—does crossfit twice a week and walks her dog two miles three times a week
- Current medications: Sumatriptan, Propranolol
- Pregnancy prevention program: abstinence—is not dating anyone at this time
- Current medical problems
  - Migraines

Social History

- She lives alone, and is a nurse in a TB clinic.
- Drinks one glass of wine each evening, she denies any illicit drug use.
- No history of use of tobacco.

PMH: Denies history of stroke, cardiovascular disease, arteriosclerosis, valvular heart disease, uncontrolled hypertension, glaucoma, hyperthyroidism, seizures, renal disease, pulmonary hypertension, or pancreatitis.

Family History: adopted with no information about her biologic parents, no known siblings.

ROS General: generally able to accomplish all activities of daily living, no change in strength or exercise tolerance. Head: + migraines, no vertigo. Eyes: Normal vision, no diplopia. Chest: No dyspnea. Heart: No chest pains, no palpitations, no syncope, no orthopnea. Abdomen: no dysphagia, no abdominal pains, no bowel habit changes, no emesis. Neurologic: No weakness, no tremor, no seizures, no changes in mentation. Psychiatric: No depressive symptoms, no changes in sleep habits, no changes in thought content. Sleep–wakes feeling rested most days. Pain—occasional back pain after crossfit.

Physical Exam

VS: BP 130/82 HR 75 RR 16 Pox 96% 5′6″ 205# BMI 33 kg/m^2

Objective General: patient in NAD, cooperative with examiner, well groomed, alert and oriented × 4.

Eyes: PERRL, Eyes: conjunctivae clear, no discharge. Ears: Canals clear bilaterally, TM's normal bilaterally. Nose: Moist, pink mucosa without lesions or mass. Throat: no exudates, no erythema.

Neck: Supple, no masses, no thyromegaly, no bruits, no lymphadenopathy.

Chest: BSCTA = bil, no rales, no rhonchi, no wheezes, speaking in full sentences, respirations non labored.

Heart/CV: RR, no rubs, no gallops; Radial and pedal pulses 2+ = bil.

Abdomen: bowel sounds normal, percussion tones nl, SNT without rebound, no masses, no splenomegaly. Liver is 14 cm at MCL on percussion and 1 cm below the costal margin.

Neuro: A&O × 4, CN II-XII grossly intact, stable gait, romberg negative, DTR's 2+ and = bilaterally, recent and distant memory grossly intact.

Extremities: Warm, well perfused, no edema, grips and pushes 2+ = bilaterally.

Screenings completed: BED- 7 SCORE: negative. STOPBANG: negative PHQ9 Score of 0 PARQ negative.

Recent labs show her CBC, TSH, FT4, FT3 are within normal range. Total cholesterol is 198, LDL is 110, triglycerides 330, HDL 38, her hemoglobin A-1 C is 5.5, CMP nl except ALT 92 u/L AST 82 u/L.

Chart Note

Diagnose and Stage

According to AACE, Susan has obesity. Her BMI is 33 kg/m^2 with a waist circumference of 40″, which represents excess visceral adiposity, and she has hypertriglyceridemia and elevated liver enzymes with liver enlargement, with minimal alcohol intake and obesity likely NALFD. These place her at diagnostic stage 2.

- Susan Miller 28 years.
- Diagnosis of obesity Stage 2 E66.8 based on BMI of 33 and ORCs.
- E78.1 Elevated triglycerides as evidenced by triglycerides 330. Will treat the elevated triglycerides with treatment of obesity at this time but monitor every 6 months.
- R94. 5 Elevated liver enzymes as evidenced by AST 82 and ALT 92, likely NALFD and will be treated with obesity but will refer to GI for full evaluation.
- G43.909 migraine.
- Met with patient for 40 minutes, completed intake history and physical examination and did education on the disease of obesity.

- No referrals needed based on screening.
- Discussed currently recommended obesity management strategies.
- Introduction to the practice, My Fitness Pal will send connection information and the importance of tracking.
- Education on obesity as a disease.
- Plan for next visit:
  - Track on My Fitness Pal
  - Patient will be monitoring intake very closely so will review this at the next visit.
  - Decision on food plan choice will be made patient was given handout on eating plan options.
  - Patient to continue existing exercise program.
  - Decrease alcohol content and avoid Tylenol containing substances—will do referral to GI for follow-up on elevated enzymes and enlarged liver.
  - Next visit in 2 weeks.

- [Practice note: In summary, Susan's evaluation demonstrates a diagnosis of obesity, migraines, new diagnosis of hypertriglycerides and suspected NALFD. She has a history of weight loss and regain. Has repeated attempts at weight loss.]This visit was coded as followsE&M 99214 – patient with provider for 40 minutes with significant history and physical
  - ICD10 E66.8
  - G47.33 Sleep apnea
  - K21.9 GERD
  - F32.2 Major Depression Disorder
  - R73.03 Prediabetes
  - E78.2 Mixed Hyperlipidemia
  - M17.9 OA, knees

	Visit Two	Visit Three
HX	Review food tracking: She is averaging 2200 calories a day, CHO ~ 325/day, PRO ~55gm/day Physical activity tracking—2 mile walks 3 days a week and crossfit 2 days a week Has not had a migraine in the past 2 weeks States received a call from GI and has an appointment later in the week	Review food tracking: She is averaging 1800 calories a day, CHO 150 g/day, Protein 90 g/day with 30 g at breakfast everyday Notices decrease of hunger through the day from weeks before but still is hungry Patient reports eating fast food five times in the past 2 weeks Review physical activity tracking—no change in activity phentermine 3.75 mg/topiramate 23 mg extended release Stopped propranolol No migraines in past 2 weeks Has stopped all alcohol Denies any side effects of Qsymia
ROS	*General*: Patient denies change in exercise tolerance. Denies insomnia *Lungs*: Patient denies SOB w usual activity and Shortness of breath at rest *Heart*: Patient denies Palpitations, Irregular heartbeat, and Chest pains *GI*: Patient denies Changes in way food taste, Dry mouth, Abdominal pain, Nausea, Vomiting, Diarrhea, and Constipation *Neurologic*: Patient denies Headache, Numbness in extremities, Dizziness, word find issues, or paresthesias *Psychiatric*: Patient denies Suicidal thoughts and Depression *Endocrine*: Patient denies Excessive thirst or hunger	*General*: Patient denies change in exercise tolerance. Denies insomnia *Lungs*: Patient denies SOB w usual activity and Shortness of breath at rest *Heart*: Patient denies Palpitations, Irregular heartbeat, and Chest pains. *GI*: Patient denies Changes in way food taste, Dry mouth, Abdominal pain, Nausea, Vomiting, Diarrhea, and Constipation *Neurologic*: Patient denies Headache, Numbness in extremities, Dizziness, word find issues, or paresthesias *Psychiatric*: Patient denies Suicidal thoughts and Depression *Endocrine*: Patient denies Excessive thirst or hunger

(continued)

	Visit Two	Visit Three
PE	VS: BP 132/82 HR 82 RR 16 pOx 98% 5′6″ 206# BMI 33 kg/m^2 Patient is alert and oriented × 4, recent and remote memory intact. Breathing is non-labored, patient speaking in full sentences. Radial pulse has RRR. Skin is normal color, cap refill is <2 seconds. Gait is normal	VS: BP 128/76 HR 84 RR 16 pOx 98% 5′6″ 200# BMI 32.28 kg/m^2 Patient is alert and oriented × 4, recent and remote memory intact. Breathing is non-labored, patient speaking in full sentences. Radial pulse has RRR. Skin is normal color, cap refill is <2 seconds. Gait is normal
DX	Diagnosis of obesity Stage 2 E66.8 based on BMI of 33 original BMI 33 and ORCs E78.1 Elevated triglycerides as evidenced by triglycerides 330. Will treat the elevated triglycerides with treatment of obesity at this time but monitor every 6 months R94. 5 Elevated liver enzymes as evidenced by AST 82 and ALT 92, likely NALFD and will be treated with obesity but will refer to GI for full evaluation G43.909 Migraine	Diagnosis of obesity Stage 2 E66.8 based on BMI of 32.28 original BMI 33 and ORCs E78.1 Elevated triglycerides as evidenced by triglycerides 330 Will treat the elevated triglycerides with treatment of obesity at this time but monitor every 6 months. K75.81 NALFD as evidenced by AST 82 and ALT 92, and based on consult note from GI referral with recommendation to treat with obesity treatment and monitor liver enzymes in 6 months—no ETOH and limited or no tylenol G43.909 Migraine

Plan	Met with patient for 25 minutes, 20 minutes in counseling and education Susan says her goal is to be less fatigued, have fewer headaches and feel more comfortable in her own skin, would like to wear a size 10 again. Goals from a health perspective goals could include eliminating or minimizing obesity related complications and comorbidities which should be seen at about 5–10% weight loss. Susan agrees with this plan Discussed eating plans and patient states would like to move to ketogenic eating plan as she has several friends that are eating this way so she would have support. Discussed with patient that going from CHO of 325 to under 30 may make her feel pretty bad initially. SMART GOAL: will limit fast food to two times a week and pack her lunch the evening before to take to work. SMART GOAL: Reduce CHO to maximum of 150 g/day Utilized current food tracking diary to demonstrate to patient where she is getting the majority of CHO so she could begin to make the decrease	Met with patient for 25 minutes, 20 minutes in counseling and education SMART goals were met—ate out 4 times at fast food over 2 weeks and packed lunch. CHO reduced to less than 150 g/day Discussed continued eating changes SMART GOAL: Reduce CHO to maximum of 100 g/day Activity plan: continue with current activity Medication management: increase to 7.5/46 mg dose of Qsymia Monitor hunger Pregnancy prevention remains in place. Patient provided with handouts on protein grams in food and protein snacks. Handouts provided on keto snacks, keto shopping Follow-up plan for this visit: Continue to Track intake on My Fitness Pal Increase Qsymia dose to 7.5 mg/46 mg tablet each morning Monitor hunger and satiety Reduce CHO to maximum of 100 g/day Follow-up appointment in 2 weeks Email or call with any concerns Education at this appointment use of protein

(continued)

	Visit Two	Visit Three
	Medication management decision: discussed medication options. Due to migraines will start phentermine/topiramate in order to potentially use topiramate to assist with migraine prevention. Placed with mail order pharmacy. Patient to start at dose of 3.75/23 and will increase dose if needed. Pregnancy prevention informed consent signed. Patient verbalized understanding of need to continue pregnancy prevention with abstinence and if she is going to start dating she will need to have a reliable pregnancy prevention plan put into place. Patient provided with medication handout, reviewed with no questions. Follow-up plan for this visit: Continue to Track intake on My Fitness Pal Track hunger and satiety (provided with handout) with start of anti-obesity medication Will stop propranolol in 2 weeks after having Qsymia on board Qsymia 3.75/23 mg to start one tab in am Follow-up appointment in 2 weeks Email or call with any concerns Education at this appointment around eating and medications	
Billing	99214 (time) ICD10 E66.8 Obesity E78.1 Elevated triglycerides R94. 5 Elevated liver enzymes G43.909 Migraine Z71.3 Dietary surveillance and counseling	99214 (time) ICD10 E66.8 Obesity E78.1 Elevated triglycerides K75.81 NALFD G43.909 Migraine Z71.3 Dietary surveillance and counseling Z71.89 Exercise counseling

	Visit Four	Visit Five	Visit Six – 22
HX	Review food tracking: She is averaging 1600 calories a day, CHO net 30 g/day for past week, Protein 80 g/day—has no fast food for past 2 weeks. Is not getting 30 g of protein at breakfast on Saturday and Sunday—says she wants 2 days a week off of shakes Notices a significant decrease of hunger Review physical activity tracking—continues with 2 mile walks 3 days a week and cross fit 2 days a week Taking Qsymia as directed—continues with abstinence Had to use rescue medication for one migraine past 2 weeks—successful in stopping headache Denies any side effects of Qsymia	Review food tracking: She is averaging 1500 calories a day, CHO 30 g/day, Protein 90 g/day until past 3 days and has been eating whatever she wants on her vacation to Santa Fe, NM. Was frustrated with lack of weight loss past 2 weeks and "Sort of gave up and figured while I was on vacation, I would just eat what I wanted" Review physical activity tracking—did same activity until vacation and has not tracked any of activity but has walked a lot Had two migraines on vacation but rescue medication was successful Taking Qsymia one tablet in am and Denies any side effects of Qsymia and continuing abstinence	Continue to review food tracking and any roadblocks with shared decision-making to get around them. Monitor medication and side effects Patient has been able to maintain her ketogenic eating plan since Visit 5 At 1 year activity continues with walking 3 days a week and crossfit 2 days a week No migraines in past 4 months Dose of Qsymia remained stable with no side effects

(continued)

	Visit Four	Visit Five	Visit Six – 22
ROS	*General*: Patient denies change in exercise tolerance. Denies insomnia *Lungs*: Patient denies SOB w usual activity and Shortness of breath at rest *Heart*: Patient denies Palpitations, Irregular heartbeat, and Chest pains *GI*: Patient denies Changes in way food taste, Dry mouth, Abdominal pain, Nausea, Vomiting, Diarrhea, and Constipation *Neurologic*: Patient denies Headache, Numbness in extremities, Dizziness, word find issues, or paresthesias *Psychiatric*: Patient denies Suicidal thoughts and Depression *Endocrine*: Patient denies Excessive thirst or hunger	*General*: Patient denies change in exercise tolerance. Denies insomnia *Lungs*: Patient denies SOB w usual activity and Shortness of breath at rest *Heart*: Patient denies Palpitations, Irregular heartbeat, and Chest pains *GI*: Patient denies Changes in way food taste, Dry mouth, Abdominal pain, Nausea, Vomiting, Diarrhea, and Constipation *Neurologic*: Patient denies Headache, Numbness in extremities, Dizziness, word find issues, or paresthesias *Psychiatric*: Patient denies Suicidal thoughts and Depression *Endocrine*: Patient denies Excessive thirst or hunger	*Continue ROS for each visit*

PE	VS: BP 118/76 HR 72 RR 16 pOx 98% 5′6″ 195# BMI 31.47 kg/m2. Patient is alert and oriented × 4, recent and remote memory intact. Breathing is non-labored, patient speaking in full sentences. Radial pulse has RRR. Skin is normal color, cap refill is <2 seconds Gait is normal. PHQ9 4	VS: BP 114/68 HR 72 RR 16 pOx 98% 5′3″ 198# BMI 31.95 kg/m^2. Patient is alert and oriented × 4, recent and remote memory intact. Breathing is non-labored, patient speaking in full sentences. Radial pulse has RRR. Skin is normal color, cap refill is <2 seconds Gait is normal. PHQ9 2	Continues visits on regular basis every 2–3 weeks End of year one VS: BP 112/68 HR 72 RR 16 pOx 98% 5′6″ 162 # Waist circumference 34" BMI 26.14 kg/m^2 Patient is alert and oriented × 4, recent and remote memory intact. Breathing is non-labored, patient speaking in full sentences. Radial pulse has RRR. Skin is normal color, cap refill is <2 seconds Gait is normal. PHQ9 2 Lipid panel tested at 1 year—all levels in normal range HgBA1C 5.2

(continued)

	Visit Four	Visit Five	Visit Six – 22
DX	Diagnosis of obesity Stage 2 E66.8 based on BMI of 31.47 original BMI 33 and ORCs E78.1 Elevated triglycerides as evidenced by triglycerides 330. Will treat the elevated triglycerides with treatment of obesity at this time but monitor every 6 months K75.81 NALFD as evidenced by AST 82 and ALT 92, and based on consult note from GI referral with recommendation to treat with obesity treatment and monitor liver enzymes in 6 months—no ETOH and limited or no tylenol G43.909 Migraine	ICD10 E66.8 Obesity based on BMI of 31.95 original BMI 33 and ORCs E78.1 Elevated triglycerides as evidenced by triglycerides 330. Will treat the elevated triglycerides with treatment of obesity at this time but monitor every 6 months K75.81 NALFD as evidenced by AST 82 and ALT 92, and based on consult note from GI referral with recommendation to treat with obesity treatment and monitor liver enzymes in 6 months—no ETOH and limited or no tylenol G43.909 Migraine	ICD10 E66.8 Obesity G43.909 Migraine Able to remove elevated triglyceride and NALFD diagnosis—successfully treated with obesity treatment

Plan	Met with patient for 25 minutes, 20 minutes in counseling and education Last SMART goal was met—eating ketogenic plan 100% of time and having 30 g of protein 5 mornings a week Discussed continued eating changes Patient will continue to utilize ketogenic eating Patient decided to have SMART goal for the next 2 weeks: remain on ketogenic eating plan Activity plan: Continue Medication management: Has met the 5% requirement to continue medication and has decrease in hunger noticed as well as fewer cravings at night. Pregnancy prevention remains in place Patient provided with handouts 50 things to do instead of snacking	Met with patient for 25 minutes, 20 minutes in counseling and education Last SMART goal was not met—discussed at length the expectations of plateaus and weight regain. Additionally reviewed the need to change eating plan if not staying on ketogenic eating 100% of the time Patient stated wanted to restart on ketogenic eating as she recognized how much better she felt eating that way SMART GOAL for next 2 weeks: 30 net grams of CHO or less daily, protein back to 80–90 g per day Discussed importance of long-term food tracking Medication management: Continue Qsymia. Pregnancy prevention remains in place Patient provided with handout Managing plateaus and slips	Throughout this time continue with education at each visit At one-year plan going forward: Continue tracking food intake Discussed the maintenance plan for ketogenic eating plan Continue and increase steps Continue anaerobic activity Continue Qsymia See patient every 3 months, unless weight regain of 5 pounds then to come in sooner

(continued)

	Visit Four	Visit Five	Visit Six – 22
	Follow-up plan for this visit: Continue to Track intake on My Fitness Pal Continue Qsymia Monitor hunger and satiety SMART goal for the next 2 weeks: remain on ketogenic eating plan Follow-up appointment in 2 weeks Email or call with any concerns Education at this appointment items to use instead of snacking	Follow-up plan for this visit: Continue to Track intake on My Fitness Pal Continue current dose of Qsymia Monitor hunger and satiety SMART goal for the next 2 weeks: 30 net g of CHO or less daily, protein back to 80–90 g per day Follow-up appointment in 2 weeks Email or call with any concerns Education at this appointment ketogenic eating "all or not at all" plateaus	
Billing	99214 (time) ICD10 E66.8 Obesity E78.1 Elevated triglycerides K75.81 NALFD G43.909 Migraine Z71.3 Dietary surveillance and counseling Z71.89 Exercise counseling	99214 (time) ICD10 E66.8 Obesity E78.1 Elevated triglycerides K75.81 NALFD G43.909 Migraine Z71.3 Dietary surveillance and counseling Z71.89 Exercise counseling	99214 (time) ICD10 E66.8 Obesity G43.909 Migraine Z71.3 Dietary surveillance and counseling Z71.89 Exercise counseling

John

John arrives at the office for a commercial drivers license (CDL) visit. He is sitting in a wide comfortable chair in the waiting room and has this month's Weight Matters from the Obesity Action Coalition among other health and outdoor magazines to choose from. The MA notes a BMI of 43 from a previous visit. She gets a measured height on the patient and the weight and VS. Then in the room explains to the patient that a new "vital sign" has been added to well visits and she will be doing a waist circumference. Today's BMI is 45 with a waist circumference of 56″. After the CDL visit John is given a brochure on obesity and treatment and recommendation to make an appointment for follow-up.

John made a FU appointment with you for obesity.

Visit One for Obesity

Patient History

- Has tried multiple times to lose weight, started gaining after college, and although he occasionally loses 20 pounds, it never stays off (Fig. 15.3).
- Has not tried any anti-obesity medications but has tried every OTC found at the local health food store.
- Current eating habits; as a truck driver eats at truck stops for most meals 5 days a week but is very interested in making a change if it will help his health.
- Current physical activity—nothing specific—"walk a lot at work unloading the truck and moving items."
- Current medications: metformin, losartan, escitalopram, pepcid daily, frequent ibuprofen.
- Current medical problems
  - Sleep apnea, reports daily use of her BiPAP
  - Gastroesophageal reflux disease that is treated with pepcid
- Knee pain and back pain takes ibuprofen and tylenol
- Depression and anxiety treated successfully with escitalopram

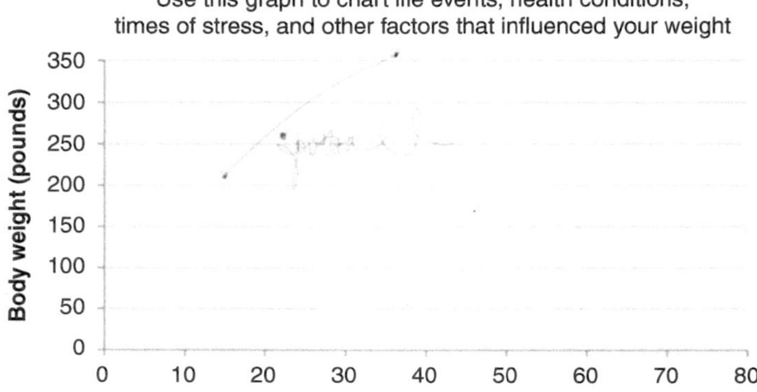

FIGURE 15.3 Body weight graph

Social History

- Lives with wife and two daughters
- Drinks socially maybe one beer per week and denies any illicit drug use
- No history of use of tobacco

PMH: Denies history of stroke, cardiovascular disease, arteriosclerosis, valvular heart disease, uncontrolled hypertension, glaucoma, hyperthyroidism, seizures, renal disease, pulmonary hypertension, or pancreatitis.

Family History: Both parents alive. "Everyone in my family is heavy" and his mother and older sister both have diabetes that came in adult years. His father has hypertension. He denies any history of cancer in the family.

ROS General: generally able to accomplish all activities of daily living, no change in strength or exercise tolerance. Head: No headaches, no vertigo. Eyes: Normal vision, no diplopia. Chest: No dyspnea. Heart: No chest pains, no palpitations, no syncope, no orthopnea. Abdomen: no dysphagia, no abdominal pains, no bowel habit changes, no emesis. Neurologic: No weakness, no tremor, no seizures, no changes in mentation. Psychiatric: No depressive symptoms, no changes in sleep habits, no changes in thought content. Sleep–wakes feeling rested when using BiPAP. Pain—occasional back and knee pain.

Physical Exam

VS: BP 138/86 HR 78 RR 16 pOx 98% 6′2″ 351# BMI 45 kg/m^2.

Objective General: patient in NAD, cooperative with examiner, well groomed, alert and oriented × 4.

Eyes: PERRL, Eyes: conjunctivae clear, no discharge. Ears: Canals clear bilaterally, TM's normal bilaterally. Nose: Moist, pink mucosa without lesions or mass. Throat: no exudates, no erythema.

Neck: Supple, no masses, no thyromegaly, no bruits, no lymphadenopathy.

Chest: BSCTA = bil, no rales, no rhonchi, no wheezes, speaking in full sentences, respirations non-labored.

Heart/CV: RR, no rubs, no gallops; Radial and pedal pulses 2+ = bil.

Abdomen: bowel sounds normal, percussion tones nl, SNT without rebound, no masses, no hepatomegaly or splenomegaly.

Neuro: A&O × 4, CN II-XII grossly intact, stable gait, romberg negative, DTR's 2+ and = bilaterally, recent and distant memory grossly intact.

Extremities: Warm, well perfused, no edema, grips and pushes 2+ = bilaterally.

Screenings completed: BED-7 SCORE: negative. STOPBANG: Not done as patient has diagnosis of Sleep Apnea PHQ9 Score of 4 PARQ negative.

Recent labs show her CMP, CBC, TSH, FT4, FT3 are within normal range. Total cholesterol is 202, LDL is 134, triglycerides 250, HDL 33, and hemoglobin A-1 C is 6.3.

Chart Note

Diagnosis and Stage

According to AACE, John has obesity. His BMI is 45 kg/m^2 with a waist circumference of 54″, which represents excess visceral adiposity, and he has several obesity-related complications (Diabetes, GERD, hyperlipidemia, osteoarthritis) and comorbidities (depression and OSA). AACE Stage 2

- John Smith 36 years old
- Diagnosis of obesity Stage 2 E66.8 based on BMI of 45 and ORCs

Due to John's BMI and 2-year history of diabetes you explain that a referral for bariatric surgery is the most appropriate treatment for him. John agrees that he would like to explore this and a referral is made to a regional bariatric surgery program. If John is not able to go to the referral OR his insurance does not have coverage, he is encouraged to return to the practice to review medical management of obesity. He leaves the practice with his referral, handout on various eating plans, and education on the importance of starting to track his food so that the bariatric program will have this information when he has his first appointment.

Practice Pearls
- Patients need frequent follow-up for this chronic disease with an intensive lifestyle intervention program.
- Each patient will need different education based on their roadblocks.
- Motivational Interviewing allows the provider to assist that patient in moving through the journey.

Conclusion

IN THE END WE COME UP WITH A CONCLUSION THAT WE NEED TO START FROM SOMEWHERE.

DEYTH BANGER

Before leaving I would like to review the updated Obesity Society statement. TOS believes that the benefits of defining obesity as a disease outweigh the commonly advanced counterarguments. One of those arguments is that excess adiposity should be viewed as an intermediate risk factor rather than as a disease. There is also the argument that "medicalizing" obesity as a disease could increase stigma and bias. But consider this statement, "Recognizing obesity as a disease neither discounts the role of the individual to manage their health nor does it take the onus off of policymakers to promote healthful food and physical activity environments. Most simply, this designation implies that as a society, we should take obesity as seriously as other behavior-related diseases that affect our collective health," Obesity Society Councilor for Advocacy/Public Affairs/Regulatory Scott Kahan, MD, FTOS, of Johns Hopkins Bloomberg School of Public Health in Baltimore, Md.

This statement combined with the information about obesity as the cause of so many diseases puts those of us in primary care in a position where we MUST treat obesity. Our

A. Golden, *Treating Obesity in Primary Care*,
https://doi.org/10.1007/978-3-030-48683-9

patients need for us to step forward and provide them with evidence-based treatment.

Evidence-based treatment includes helping patients change their eating, increasing their physical activity, and using intensive lifestyle intervention to guide the patients' journey while assuring that they can get medications as appropriate and/or referral for surgical interventions. The evidence is clear that this treatment requires frequent contact with an ILI program of some sort, whether in a primary care office or an interdisciplinary program.

As a primary care provider we are often thought of as "the jack of all trades and the master of none." I would suggest that this disease is one we must become the master of as 70% of Americans either have preobesity or obesity and that number is only growing.

Thank you for your interest in helping patients with obesity. As a person with obesity and for all the people with obesity I have known we appreciate providers that understand the disease of obesity and are willing to partner with us to control the disease, its impact on our quality of life, and all the diseases it can cause.

Resources

- https://obesitymedicine.org/obesity-algorithm/.
- http://www.obesityaction.org/educational-resources/brochures-and-guides.
- https://www.aace.com/sites/all/files/Obesity_Guidelines_Algorithm_slides_FINAL_2016.pdf.
- http://www.obesity.org/publications/obesity-journal/patient-pages.
- Treating Obesity in Primary Care Course: see https://npobesitytreatment.org for more information.

- Introduction to Obesity Management in Primary Care from AANP: https://aanp.inreachce.com/Details/Information/b6cbae97-1a16-451b-a30e-a6d713bc52d1.
- ASMBS post op guideline: As we look at the vitamins that need monitored it is easy to see why anemia can occur, especially pernicious anemia. For more detailed explanation and understanding of the complete follow-up the ASMBS has a guideline to assist (ASMBS 2013). https://asmbs.org/resources/clinical-practice-guidelines-for-the-perioperative-nutritional-metabolic-and-nonsurgical-support-of-the-bariatric-surgery-patient.

Index

A. Golden, *Treating Obesity in Primary Care*,
https://doi.org/10.1007/978-3-030-48683-9

P

R